Global Health Leadership and Management

William H. Foege
Nils Daulaire
Robert E. Black
Clarence E. Pearson
Editors

Foreword by
David Rockefeller

· ·

Global Health Leadership and Management

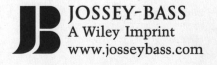

JOSSEY-BASS
A Wiley Imprint
www.josseybass.com

Published by Jossey-Bass
A Wiley Imprint
989 Market Street, San Francisco, CA 94103-1741   www.josseybass.com

Jossey-Bass books and products are available through most bookstores. To contact Jossey-Bass directly call our Customer Care Department within the U.S. at 800-956-7739, outside the U.S. at 317-572-3986, or fax 317-572-4002.

Jossey-Bass also publishes its books in a variety of electronic formats. Some content that appears in print may not be available in electronic books.

Library of Congress Cataloging-in-Publication Data

Global health leadership and management / William H. Foege ... [et al.], editors ; foreword by David Rockefeller.— 1st ed.
    p. ; cm.
Includes bibliographical references and index.
ISBN-13 978-0-7879-7153-3
ISBN-10 0-7879-7153-7 (alk. paper)
1. World health. 2. Medical policy. 3. Health services administration.
[DNLM: 1. Health Services Administration. 2. World Health. 3. Health Policy.
4. International Cooperation. 5. Leadership.] I. Foege, William H., 1936-
RA441.G5685 2005
362.1—dc22   2005003187

Printed in the United States of America
FIRST EDITION
HB Printing   10 9 8 7 6 5 4 3 2 1

Contents

About the Global Health Council   xi

Foreword   xiii
David Rockefeller

Preface   xv
William H. Foege

Acknowledgments   xxvii

Editors   xxix

Contributors   xxxi

Part One: Identifying Challenges and Developing and Managing Policy

1. First Annual Gates Award for Global Health 3
Melinda French Gates

2. A New Role for Corporate America: 9
Partners in Global Health and Development
Raymond V. Gilmartin

3. From Challenges to Policy 25
Lee Jong-wook

4. Managing Health, Health Care, and Aging 37
William D. Novelli

Part Two: Developing Strategies, New Pathways, and Solutions

5. Leadership, Equity, and Global Health   55
   Harlan Cleveland

6. HIV/AIDS: Lessons from Brazil   75
   Susan Dentzer

7. Corruption and Health Care: 93
   Need for New Solutions
   Peter Eigen

8. Business Approach to HIV/AIDS   103
   Crisis in Africa
   Spencer T. King

9. Health in the Developing World: 113
   Achieving the Millennium
   Development Goals
   Jeffrey D. Sachs

Part Three: Creating Networks and Partnerships and Planning Change from Within

10. Leadership and Management for Improving   123
    Global Health
    Frances Hesselbein

11. Creating Public Health Alliances: 129
    The American Cancer Society Experience
    John R. Seffrin

Part Four: Learning from Experience and Building a Generation of Leaders

12. Leadership Development for Global Health   147
    Jo Ivey Boufford

13. Challenges to Health in Eastern Europe   167
and the Former Soviet Union: A Decade
of Experience
Martin McKee

14. Building the Next Generation of Leaders   187
Joy Phumaphi

15. Creating Public Health Leaders: Public   201
Health Leadership Institutes
William L. Roper and Janet Porter

Part Five: Leading and Managing Teams While Recognizing and Celebrating Success

16. Leading for Success   217
Nils Daulaire

17. Epilogue: The Road Ahead   227
Kofi A. Annan

Index   229

About the Global Health Council

. . . .

The Global Health Council (GHC) is the world's largest membership alliance dedicated to advancing policies and programs that improve health around the world. Now in its twenty-ninth year, GHC has built a global coalition that promotes improvement and equity in health for all the world's citizens. It promotes better health by assuring access to essential information and resources for all who work to improve global health.

GHC is an umbrella organization composed of professionals in the health care field, nongovernmental and governmental organizations, academic institutions, foundations, and corporations. GHC serves its members and promotes equity in health through advocacy, building global alliances, and communicating experiences and best practices.

Five Key Issues

The Global Health Council is a not-for-profit organization established in 1971 as the National Council for International Health. GHC focuses on five key issues, which reflect the major contributors to the global burden of ill health:

- Child Health
- HIV/AIDS

- Reproductive and Maternal Health

- Infectious Diseases

- Emerging Global Health Threats

As a vehicle for informed and effective advocacy, GHC works to raise the priority of health issues among the American public, Congress and the Administration, international and domestic government agencies, academic institutions, and the global health community.

GHC strikes a balance between acknowledging work that needs to be done and celebrating and promoting successful programs, policies, and other initiatives that are a reality throughout the world. For more about the Global Health Council, visit their Web site at www.globalhealth.org.

Foreword

. . . .

Severe acute respiratory syndrome (SARS); mad cow disease; the HIV/AIDS (human immunodeficiency virus–acquired immunodeficiency syndrome) pandemic; obesity "epidemics" in the United States and Western Europe; the emergence of drug-resistant strains of malaria and tuberculosis in Africa, Asia, and Latin America. This ominous list of new diseases, old diseases in recombined forms, and food-based and environmental threats to human health may be only the tip of the iceberg. Just at the time when the biomedical sciences are pushing back the frontiers of molecular biology and genetics—advances that hold promise of lengthening human life expectancy to well beyond a hundred years—we seem to be losing ground in many other areas of human health. It looks as if the human race's ancient microbial enemies may once again be gaining the upper hand. Unless, that is, something is done quickly and effectively to reverse these alarming trends.

Our contemporary health crisis results from the convergence of a number of factors. There are three to which I would assign particular importance. The first is the rapid growth in world population. Now at six billion and counting, the human race is crowded into ever-denser concentrations, especially sprawling "megacities" such as Mexico City, Calcutta, Shanghai, and a dozen others scattered across the globe. In addition to making contagion easier to transmit, population increase has placed unprecedented pressure on food supplies, sources of potable water, and basic infrastructure systems everywhere. The second factor is the increasing integration of the world's economic, financial, transportation, and communications systems. The processes of integration, which we now call "globalization," have gradually gained speed and increased in intensity over the past two centuries. Along with its many significant benefits, globalization has now clearly outstripped the ability of our institutions, especially governments, to regulate and intelligently manage the flow of capital, people, and viruses across national boundaries. The final factor is the diminished capacity of governments to respond to new challenges. Not only have the effectiveness and efficacy of government been called into question in recent years, governments are also caught in a severe funding trap. This is especially notable in the nations of the developed world, where the need to fund entitlements—pensions and health care in particular—has collided head on with demands for lower tax rates. One of the casualties has been discretionary funding for public health programs.

What we can and must do to manage the looming public health crisis around the world is precisely the subject of *Global Health Leadership and Management*. William H. Foege has brought together an impressive group of individuals who have written compellingly about the need for action, especially in finding and training a new generation of leaders to resolve the massive threats that now confront us. I enthusiastically recommend this book to professionals in the field of public health, policymakers, politicians, and anyone concerned about the health, prosperity, and well-being of future generations. We can rebuild our public health systems, and we need to do it immediately. This book will help show the way.

February 2005

David Rockefeller
New York

Preface

Practitioners of global health have ever-evolving definitions of the field. For many, it was in the past known as "international health," and that in turn was synonymous with "tropical medicine." Later it came to mean health problems in tropical areas and then health problems of poor countries. It is indeed more than tropical medicine, as shown by the fact that the most lethal agent in the developing world has moved from the measles virus two decades ago (a global problem and not limited to the tropics) to tobacco use in the twenty-first century. Although the focus is certainly on the health problems of poor countries, most have dropped the title of international health in favor of "global health" to avoid a polarization of international versus national. The health problems of both rich and poor countries are so intertwined that they must be understood as a unity, but the emphasis in this book is how to make a global approach to health result in improvements of the health of poor people in poor countries.

Most books about global health in the past concentrated on the unique science involved with the life cycles of tropical parasites or the tools available to respond to these problems. In this book, we want to look at the interface of traditional global health books with the many lessons available from the field of management and the rich experience that has been gathered by those who have implemented a variety of programs in the field. How could we incorporate the experience of the for-profit field to improve the return on investment as measured by morbidity and mortality?

What has happened in global health that leads to this moment where the lack of management skills appears to be the single most important barrier to improving health throughout the world?

Participants in Global Health

The history of any endeavor is like a condensed book that we open in the middle. Our understanding is incomplete, and whereas it is apparent that every development is built on earlier activities, the early forces in the history are often unknown. That is certainly true regarding our knowledge of global health. Early health knowledge was shared between countries and regions more by the diffusion of general knowledge than through organized medical efforts. Greek and Roman experience in science and medicine became global as it became part of the knowledge soaked up by the early Islamic intellectual sponge, which was involved in seeking knowledge, including converting Greek manuscripts to Arabic. Later, when many Greek writings were lost, the knowledge of Greek science was recirculated back to Europe when the Arabic documents were translated to Latin. Modern global health efforts have been more deliberate and owe tribute to a series of events.

One force in global health resulted from the role of faith groups in organizing efforts to bring the science of Europe and the United States to developing countries. Whereas some of the early efforts were inspired by the desire to keep missionaries healthy, it soon became apparent that the local populations benefited from the skills of medical personnel. Not surprisingly, such benefits often led to the medical work becoming intertwined with proselytizing.

By the early twentieth century, medical mission work was being conducted throughout Africa, Asia, and South America. By midcentury some groups, especially the Catholic Church, had started a movement to make medical work an expression of beliefs rather than a tool for conversion. With the help of the Christian Medical Commission of the World Council of Churches, this approach had become the accepted approach for most faith groups at century's end. Whereas early efforts often found various faith groups feeling competitive with other faith groups, the Christian Medical Commission was surprisingly effective in promoting community approaches: it urged cooperation with other faith groups and influenced faith groups to coordinate their work under the umbrella of government supervision.

The efforts of faith groups had several profound effects. First, many Americans learned of the health needs of the world through communications from these medical missionaries. Second, the efforts provided a tradition of Americans and Europeans choosing career paths in global health, a practice that continued to provide many recruits for nonfaith groups, even when secular organizations took over much of the effort. Third, training programs were started for indigenous health workers, and in some places, such as India, church-sponsored medical schools became the gold standard of medical training programs for the entire country. Fourth, medical missionaries would often focus on problems such as leprosy that received a paucity of attention from country and colonial officers.

A second force involved the military. Much of the research on tropical diseases that has been sponsored by the United States is the result of military efforts to protect its own personnel when they serve in tropical areas. The findings, whether involving an understanding of basic life cycles, antimalarial drugs and other medications, or experience in clinical care, quickly found their way into civilian use. Even the Centers for Disease Control and Prevention (CDC) had its origin in a malaria control program developed in Atlanta in 1942. Military recruits who were sent from all parts of the country to the South for training were acquiring malaria. A program was instituted for malaria control, with the first objective being a one-mile mosquito-free barrier around every military installation. After the war, this program was converted to become the Communicable Disease Center, which evolved to CDC.

A third important factor throughout the twentieth century was the work of the Rockefeller Foundation. The foundation has pioneered work in hookworm control, public health education, and medical training in China and other Asian countries and later throughout the world. With emphasis on the neglected diseases of mankind, the Rockefeller Foundation has left a legacy in both the research community and the public health delivery community that has made global health an acceptable career path for a small number of individuals.

Although the accumulation of global health programs has been great because of nongovernmental organizations and many university programs, it was the growth of global health agencies and bilateral health programs after the Second World War that began to accelerate the development of global health efforts. The work of the United Nations Children's Fund (UNICEF) led over the decades to a concerted effort to improve child health in every country. Priorities were selected, resources obtained, and standards developed for immunization, oral rehydration, and a variety of programs that have reduced morbidity and mortality, especially for children younger than five. The World Health Organization (WHO) provided a framework for developing standards, technical guidelines, strategies for disease control, and both eradication and control programs for dozens of disease conditions and a forum for global debate on priorities and interventions.

Bilateral health assistance programs by the United States, Canada, and European countries matured in the second half of the twentieth century. They have involved a wide spectrum of activities— from infrastructure development to immunization programs, eradication programs, family planning and population activities, and training programs both in and out of country. Just as faith-based health programs had to overcome a tendency to use health work as a proselytizing tool, so have bilateral programs had to resist the tendency to use health for political purposes. And just as faith-based programs had to learn to overcome competitive urges and cooperate with other denominations, so have bilateral programs had to learn the value of cooperating with other countries and global agencies. It is a lesson yet to be fully learned.

Other participants include a host of nongovernmental agencies, many foundations, academic institutions, faith-based agencies, and also special-issue groups focused on a disease, on orphans, or on a specific intervention. Some provide equipment, some provide animals, and others provide a specific drug or vaccine. Many organizations target microfinancing for poor people, education programs of all kinds, and development projects. All of these programs have an effect on improving health. In sum, these thousands of agencies involve hundreds of thousands of people, and the net effect is a major impact on global health and global health activities.

Global Health Tools

As the number of participants has grown, so have the tools that can affect the health of people. Fifty years ago, not even polio vaccine was available. Vaccines have now become the foundation of global health programs: they have a great return on investment, can provide lifetime protection, and although they require all of the ingredients of a public health program—including surveillance, logistics, delivery systems, and evaluation—they are generally less complex than most public health programs and become natural entry points for the development of public health. The routine immunization schedule now includes diphtheria, pertussis, tetanus vaccine, BCG vaccine, poliomyelitis, measles, and hepatitis B vaccine. In some areas, the administration of yellow fever vaccine and *Haemophilus influenzae* type B vaccine are standard. In the next fifty years, a dozen vaccines will be available to be given, and another dozen will be used in specific areas. Heat-stable vaccines will reduce the complexity of delivery, and needles and syringes will no longer be required. Combinations of vaccines will reduce the number of doses given, and most vaccines will be effective if given shortly after birth. Adverse reactions will be increasingly rare.

The development of an array of tools to provide couples a choice on child spacing has been one of the important chapters in global health. The regulation of ovulation by means of hormonal drugs, along with condoms, intrauterine devices, diaphragms, and other tools, has provided choices to people who in the past had fatalistically accepted their lot. Simply spacing children can lead to better health even if the number of children borne by a woman remains the same. Global health and reproductive choices are inextricably linked. The devaluation of either leads to needless suffering.

The development of drugs that can be used on a mass basis with relatively few side effects has been a welcomed change in global health. Mectizan (ivermectin) changed the approach to global health when introduced in 1987 for the treatment of river blindness. Early uses were measured and gradual to detect adverse effects as a larger number of people were exposed to the drug. Widespread use has now shown it to be one of the safest drugs ever used, and by 2002, more than 250 million treatments had been given in Africa. The mass use of albendazole for lymphatic filariasis, zithromax for trachoma, and praziquantel for schistosomiasis are examples of how corporations in the past fifteen years have changed the approaches to global health.

A host of other examples, such as heat-sensitive labels on polio vaccine to determine the cold chain history; better, faster, and less expensive diagnostic techniques that can be used in the field; inexpensive prosthesis; and mass eye surgery approaches all show the exploding ability to bring science and technology to bear on global health. Perhaps no example is as fundamental as the ability to communicate. Computers and the Internet have permitted rapid sharing of information and made it possible for workers in many parts of the world to lose their isolation. Whereas telemedicine and the transmission of x-ray images are dramatic, the basic ability to com-

municate by e-mail and to obtain copies of recent articles and
reports has made it possible for field workers to truly be part of a
global team.

Global Health Resources

Global health has always been compromised by institutionalized
poverty. Inadequate resources will forever be a concern for global
health workers, but a marked difference has been apparent in the
past two decades. One change was initiated by the decision of Rotary
International in 1985 to support the global eradication of polio.
The amount of resources raised—over $500 million (U.S.) to date—
is significant. Even more significant has been the interest of an influential group of Rotarians around the world in a health problem.
Rotary money is new money to global health that does not require
the reallocation of money that would have gone to some other global
health problem. This has helped to provide credibility to the field.

The second important development was the formation of the
Bill and Melinda Gates Foundation. Again, the money was new to
global health and has given courage and hope to those who have
spent their lives in the field. The money has helped to increase
research for tools of special need in poor countries. Interestingly,
putting money into the search for new vaccines, better vaccines,
diagnostic tools for remote clinics, better drugs for tuberculosis, and
so on has increased the flow of resources into such areas from other
agencies rather than simply replacing resources from other agencies.
Also, the interest of schools of public health in global health has
dramatically increased: in some schools, such as Emory University
in Atlanta, the international health track is the greatest source of
new students. When the history of global health is written a century from now, it will be clear that the catalyst for global health
equity was two people, Bill and Melinda Gates.

These two developments have had a marked effect on increased
funding from governments for approaches such as the Global

Alliance for Vaccines and Immunization and the Global Fund for AIDS (acquired immunodeficiency syndrome), tuberculosis, and malaria. Resources for global health research have also increased, as has support for a wide spectrum of global health field activities.

Global Health Interest

The fear of bioterrorism and new interest in emerging infections, including drug-resistant tuberculosis, have led to an understanding that both problems require better routine public health structures. This new understanding has led to the conclusion that an adequate defense is built on a strong domestic public health system. That, in turn, has improved the ties between traditional public health and global health. Also, economists have increased interest in global health since a report in 1993 by the World Bank highlighted the relationship between health and development. Activist economists, such as one of the contributors to this volume, Jeffrey D. Sachs of Columbia University, have promoted increased investments in global health as an important part of improving general development.

This, in turn, has led to an increase in the political interest in global health at every level. The United Nations, including Secretary-General Kofi Annan, has been involved in polio, maternal-child health, AIDS, tuberculosis, and malaria in a way that has no precedent. Former heads of state such as President Carter, General Toure of Mali, and General Gowan of Nigeria and also current heads of state now make health part of their daily agenda and their campaign promises. Global and bilateral funds are increasing, movie and music stars are becoming involved, and corporations have changed their investments in health. Merck and Company, Inc., has now given free more than three hundred million treatments for river blindness and has made a major investment in approaches to the treatment of AIDS in Botswana. GlaxoSmithKline provides a drug for lymphatic filariasis, and Pfizer has provided an antibiotic for the treatment of trachoma.

More important than each specific expression of interest has been the tendency to form coalitions of public and private groups to attack specific problems such as polio, river blindness, AIDS, tuberculosis, micronutrient malnutrition, trachoma, birth defects, tobacco use, and cervical cancer.

Much of this new interest is based on a demonstration that some things actually work and success is possible. But once again, fear has also played a role in promoting global health interest. The military interest was driven by the fear of compromised fighting strength due to diseases of the tropics. Now the fear of AIDS, multidrug-resistant tuberculosis, malaria, avian influenza, severe acute respiratory syndrome (SARS), and other diseases has led governments to take a new interest in finding solutions.

Global Health Skills

Early global health work looked to the skills of medical practitioners. Medical missionaries ran clinics and hospitals, but even the promotion of public health programs relied heavily on physicians. It is now apparent that the skills of planning, developing surveillance systems, analyzing data, using epidemiological findings, organizing logistics systems, delivering products, and evaluating results are even more important than medical or scientific skills. Increasingly, the field looks to problem solvers, managers, and people who know how to get things done. There is also new appreciation of the social sciences: they have always been important in public health, but the AIDS pandemic has reminded the field anew of the importance of anthropologists, sociologists, psychologists, and ethicists.

The Challenge

Management has always been important in global health. The difference between a body of scientific knowledge making a difference in improving suffering and postponing death comes down to delivery or the use of that knowledge. That is the big gap in global health. Donations of free drugs or vaccines are useless if the system is not capable of getting them to those in need. That is the challenge of this book.

Immunization programs improved rapidly in the 1980s. In 1984, less than 15 percent of children in the world were getting measles vaccine—this despite the fact that it was a relatively inexpensive vaccine and that the measles virus was the single most lethal agent in the world. In March of that year, UNICEF, WHO, the World Bank, the United Nations Development Programme, and the Rockefeller Foundation organized a Task Force for Child Survival to see whether coordinated approaches could improve basic immunization coverage. Six years later, UNICEF reported that 80 percent of children in the world were receiving basic immunizations, including measles vaccine. Jim Grant, executive director of UNICEF, said it was the single greatest peacetime achievement the world had ever seen.

Not to downplay the difficulty of delivering immunizations, it is easier to do that than to find and treat all people with tuberculosis or to set up a system that effectively provides rehydration fluid for all children with diarrhea. And yet, achieving a level of 80 percent immunization coverage was not sufficiently motivating to inspire countries to maintain the effort. Immunization levels gradually dropped in the 1990s, especially in Africa, and to very low levels in some countries like Nigeria.

If a country is unable to maintain an immunization program for six vaccines, it is not likely the country will do so for twelve vaccines. The great challenge is to develop immunization infrastructures that are simple and sustainable and have incentives that improve as the program improves—to develop an infrastructure worthy of what the researchers develop.

As the contributors to this book point out, science is not enough, good intentions do not change the health picture, and resources are easily wasted. We need the same constant attention that is absolutely expected in the business community, with a focus on developing objectives, working out strategies for reaching those objectives, organizing all components of a program to pursue the strategy, pushing for continuous quality improvement, and developing the ability to measure both process and outcome goals for constant midcourse corrections.

As immunization programs in the United States improved, a spectrum of results could be expected across three thousand counties. Some programs were very good, and some were an embarrassment. But it became clear that a state with lagging programs could be improved within months simply by acquiring an immunization manager who had demonstrated results in another state. Immunization leadership and management was the key, not science. There are no inherent reasons why some countries should be able to protect their children and other countries must remain vulnerable. The only two barriers are the mobilization of resources and the actual delivery of our science capacity. This comes down to creative and efficient management. Global health waits expectantly for management to match its science.

February 2005

William H. Foege
Seattle

Acknowledgments

It is difficult to thank so many individuals who made this book come to fruition, from the initial concept to its final form. Three extraordinarily talented and dedicated people who were instrumental in moving through the myriad logistics need to be recognized. First, I want to give particular and special thanks to Laurie Norris, our managing editor, who had general oversight of the project and worked with zeal, commitment, and exemplary professionalism, bringing all of the necessary components together that made this final publication possible. Second, thanks go to Andy Pasternack, Health Editor for Jossey-Bass/John Wiley & Sons, Inc., who enthusiastically supported this second volume in the global health series to build on the success of the first in the series, *Critical Issues in Global Health*. I appreciate his long experience in publishing that he brings to this volume and the professional support of his staff, particularly Seth Schwartz. Third, it is with great gratitude that I thank Clarence E. Pearson for shouldering all of the difficulties in getting drafts written, reviewed, and revised. He has a passion for sharing the world of global health.

This book on global health leadership and management came to be because nineteen recognized global leaders voluntarily shared their long and extraordinary international experiences. Each of them accepted, with no reservations, the challenge to participate as an author. Heartfelt thanks go to each of them for their thought-ful and thought-provoking contributions.

Finally, I express my deep appreciation to Robert E. Black and the Global Health Council (Nils Daulaire and associates), whose resources and connections with key leadership were instrumental in shaping this book.

W.H.F.

Editors

• •

William H. Foege, M.D., M.P.H., is senior medical advisor for the Bill and Melinda Gates Foundation. He is Presidential Distinguished Professor of International Health at the Rollins School of Public Health, Emory University in Atlanta. He served as director for the Centers for Disease Control and Prevention from 1977 to 1983 and then as the executive director of the Carter Center and the executive director of the Task Force for Child Survival and Development.

Nils Daulaire, M.D., M.P.H., is president and chief executive officer of the Global Health Council, the world's largest membership alliance dedicated to advancing policies and programs to improve health throughout the world. He has worked for two decades in health care in developing countries and served as the deputy assistant administrator for policy and program coordination at the United States Agency for International Development. A Phi Beta Kappa and summa cum laude graduate of Harvard College, Boston, Daulaire received his medical degree from Harvard Medical School and his master's in public health from Johns Hopkins University in Baltimore. He is a member of the National Academy of Science's Institute of Medicine.

Robert E. Black, M.D., M.P.H., is the Edgar Berman Professor and Chair of the Department of International Health of the Johns

Hopkins University Bloomberg School of Public Health. Dr. Black is trained in internal medicine, preventive medicine, infectious diseases, and epidemiology. He has served as a medical epidemiologist at the U.S. Centers for Disease Control and worked at institutions in Bangladesh and Peru on research related to childhood infectious diseases and nutritional problems. He is also involved in the use of evidence in policy and programs, the development of research capacity, and the strengthening of public health leadership in developing countries.

Clarence E. Pearson, M.S.P.H., is senior advisor to the World Health Organization Office at the United Nations. He was formerly president and chief executive officer of the National Center for Health Education and served as vice president of the Peter Drucker Foundation for Nonprofit Management and vice president and director of health and safety for Metropolitan Life Insurance Company. Pearson conceived and serves as executive editor of a series of books on global health published by Jossey-Bass. Along with C. Everett Koop, M.D., he coedited the first in the series, *Critical Issues in Global Health.*

Contributors

Kofi A. Annan is the seventh secretary-general of the United Nations and the first to be appointed from the ranks of United Nations staff. A national of Ghana, he joined the U.N. system in 1962 and has served the organization at headquarters and in the field, dealing with matters ranging from personnel and budget to refugee assistance and peace keeping. As secretary-general, his priorities have been to adapt the United Nations for the twenty-first century through a comprehensive program of reform; to strengthen its work for peace and development, particularly in Africa; to advocate for human rights and the rule of law; to raise global awareness of the AIDS epidemic; and to bring the United Nations closer to the public by working more closely with nongovernmental organizations, parliamentarians, academic institutions, the private sector, and other partners. After receiving his undergraduate degree in economics from Macalester College, Saint Paul, Minnesota, he did postgraduate work at the Institute of International Affairs in Geneva and as a Sloan Fellow in management at the Massachusetts Institute of Technology. Annan is married to Nane Annan of Sweden.

Jo Ivey Boufford, M.D., professor of public service, health policy, and management at the Robert F. Wagner Graduate School of Public Service at New York University and clinical professor of pediatrics at New York University Medical School, has also served as dean of the Wagner School. Previously she was principal deputy assistant secretary for health in the U.S. Department of Health and Human Services and acting assistant secretary; she concurrently served as the U.S. representative on the executive board of WHO. She is a member of the Institute of Medicine and serves on its executive council and board on global health.

Harlan Cleveland, political scientist and public executive, is president emeritus of the World Academy of Art and Science. A graduate of Princeton University in Princeton, New Jersey, and a Rhodes Scholar at Oxford in the 1930s, he has been an aid administrator in Europe and China, a Marshall Plan executive, a magazine editor and publisher, dean of two graduate schools of public affairs (at Syracuse, New York, and University of Minnesota), and president of the University of Hawaii. During the 1960s, he served as assistant secretary of state for international organization affairs under President John F. Kennedy and as United States Ambassador to NATO under President Lyndon Johnson. He is author of twelve books on international affairs and executive leadership.

Susan Dentzer since 1998 has been an on-air correspondent for the Public Broadcasting System's *NewsHour with Jim Lehrer*. She leads a unit providing in-depth coverage of health policy. Previously Dentzer was chief economics correspondent at *U.S. News & World Report* and a senior writer at *Newsweek*. A former Harvard Nieman Fellow, Dentzer was a Japan Society Leadership Fellow and in 1991 conducted research on Japan's aging population. Dentzer serves on the board of the Global Health Council and Japan Society of New York. A graduate of Dartmouth College in Hanover, New Hampshire, Dentzer served on Dartmouth's board of trustees from 1993 to 2004 and was the first female board chair.

Peter Eigen is the founder and chair of the board of Transparency International, a Berlin-based organization promoting openness and accountability in international trade and development. He studied law and economics at the universities of Erlangen/Nuremberg and Frankfurt and received a doctoral degree in law at the latter institution in 1965. In 1968, he became an attorney at the World Bank, specializing in international trade and procurement. He served as a special advisor to the governments of Botswana (1973–1974) and Namibia (1991), focusing on economic development. From the mid-1970s to the early 1990s, he managed the World Bank programs in East and West Africa and Latin America.

Melinda French Gates is cofounder of the Bill and Melinda Gates Foundation, which seeks to improve people's lives by bringing advances in health and learning to those who need them most. She works with local, national, and international partners and foundation grantees to further the foundation's goal of improving equity in four areas: global health, education, access to digital information through public libraries, and support for at-risk families in Washington and Oregon. Gates is a former member of the board of trustees of Duke University, Durham, North Carolina, and was formerly a cochair of the Washington State Governor's Commission on Early Learning.

Raymond V. Gilmartin is chair, president, and chief executive officer (CEO) of Merck & Company, Inc. Before joining Merck in 1994, he was chair, president, and CEO of Becton Dickinson and Company. He serves on the boards of directors of General Mills, Inc., and the Microsoft Corporation. He is the president of the International Federation of Pharmaceutical Manufacturers Associations and also serves on the executive committee of the Pharmaceutical Research and Manufacturers of America. Gilmartin is a member of the President's Export Council and also serves as a member of the Trans Atlantic Business Dialogue and the Trade and Poverty Forum.

Frances Hesselbein is the chair of the board of governors of the Leader To Leader Institute, formerly the Peter Drucker Foundation.

In 1998, she was awarded the Presidential Medal of Freedom, the United States of America's highest civilian honor. In 2002, Hesselbein was the first recipient of the Dwight D. Eisenhower National Security Series Award for her service with the U.S. Army. She is the author of *Hesselbein on Leadership* (2002), and with General Eric K. Shinseki, she coauthored the introduction to *Be, Know, Do: Leadership the Army Way* (2004).

Lee Jong-wook, M.D., is director-general of the World Health Organization (WHO). Before his election to this post in July 2003, he was director of the WHO Stop TB department, which includes the Stop TB Partnership, a global public-private alliance of over 250 partners. His earlier responsibilities in WHO included directing the Global Programme for Vaccines and Immunization, leading the polio eradication effort in the Western Pacific Region, and serving as Regional Adviser on Chronic Diseases. Lee, who is from the Republic of Korea, joined WHO as a leprosy consultant in the South Pacific in 1983.

Spencer T. King has more than thirty-three years' experience in international business and development and twenty-five years' experience as the director of large, multifaceted projects funded by the U.S. Agency for International Development (USAID) that offer business development services to small and medium-sized enterprises in many countries. King joined International Executive Service Corps (IESC) in 1992 and has served as chief of party for some of USAID's most successful programs, including the Technology Initiative for the Private Sector program in Sri Lanka and the Center for Business project in Egypt. He was appointed president and CEO of IESC in October 2003.

Martin McKee, M.D., M.S.C., F.R.C.P., is professor of European public health at the London School of Hygiene and Tropical Medicine, where he directs the school's European Centre of Health of Societies in Transition. He is also a research director of the

European Observatory on Health Care Systems and an editor of the *European Journal of Public Health*. Since 1990 he has been involved in many developments in public health training in the former communist countries of Central and Eastern Europe and sits on the boards of public health schools in Russia, Hungary, and Croatia. In 2003 he received the Andrija Stampar medal for his contributions to European public health.

William D. Novelli is executive director and CEO of AARP (formerly the American Association of Retired Persons), a membership organization of over thirty-five million people aged fifty and older. Before joining AARP, he was president of the Campaign for Tobacco-Free Kids and executive vice president of CARE. He cofounded and was president of Porter Novelli, an international marketing and public relations agency founded to apply marketing to social and health issues. He is a recognized leader in the international emergence of social marketing; has written extensively on marketing management, marketing communications, and social marketing; and has been recognized as one of the one hundred most influential public relations professionals of the twentieth century.

Joy Phumaphi, B. Comm, Msc., is the assistant director-general of the Family and Community Health Cluster at WHO in Geneva. She was the minister of health in Botswana until July 2003. She is a Distinguished African American Institute Fellow and is a commissioner of the U.N. Secretary-General's commission on HIV/AIDS and Governance in Africa. Phumaphi is patron of several Botswanan nongovernmental organizations dealing with children, violence, women, and human immunodeficiency virus and acquired immunodeficiency syndrome. She has served as a member of the U.N. Reference Group on Economics and on the advisory board for the United Nations Development Programme in Africa.

Janet Porter, Ph.D., is associate dean of the School of Public Health, University of North Carolina at Chapel Hill. Previously she was a hospital administrator and health care consultant for twenty years. She serves on the board of the National Center for Healthcare Leadership and the Accrediting Commission for Education in Health Services Administration.

William L. Roper, M.D., M.P.H., is vice-chancellor of medical affairs and the dean of the medical school at the University of North Carolina at Chapel Hill. He has served as the administrator of the Healthcare Financing Administration, now known as the Center for Medicare and Medicaid Services. He also served as the director of the Centers for Disease Control and Prevention in Atlanta, as senior vice president of Prudential Health Care, and as dean of the University of North Carolina School of Public Health.

Jeffrey D. Sachs is director of the Earth Institute at Columbia University in New York and special advisor to United Nations Secretary-General Kofi Annan on the Millennium Development Goals. In 2000–2001, Sachs chaired the Commission on Macroeconomics and Health for WHO. He is internationally renowned for advising governments in Latin America, Eastern Europe, the former Soviet Union, Asia, and Africa on economic reforms and for his work with international agencies to promote poverty reduction, disease control, and debt reduction of poor countries. He was recently named among the one hundred most influential leaders in the world by *Time Magazine*.

John R. Seffrin, Ph.D., has been CEO of the American Cancer Society for more than a decade. He was a charter member of the National Dialogue on Cancer, an appointee to the National Cancer Policy Board, and cochair of the National Cancer Legislation Advisory Board. He led the creation of the National Center for Tobacco-Free Kids and was appointed to the President's Commission on Improving Economic Opportunities in Communities Dependent on Tobacco Production While Protecting Public Health. Seffrin currently serves as president of the International Union Against Cancer and as chair of the board of Independent Sector.

Global Health Leadership and Management

Part I

. . . .

Identifying Challenges and
Developing and Managing Policy

. . . .

First Annual Gates Award
for Global Health

Melinda French Gates

M any people have thanked me for what the Bill and Melinda Gates Foundation is doing. Let me set the record straight. I want to thank the health workers of the world who actually apply the tools to improve the health of children around the world.

Nothing matters more to the future of our world than the well-being of women and children. If we want healthy economies, we need healthy families. If we want peaceful societies, we need peaceful communities. If we want a meaningful standard of human rights, then we have to uphold women's rights and children's rights.

In 1941, Franklin D. Roosevelt helped make human rights more concrete when he spelled out the four freedoms that unified Americans at a dark moment in our history:

- Freedom of speech

- Freedom of worship

The Gates Award was developed to acknowledge organizations that have made a lasting contribution to global health by actually changing health. It rewards not simply the science but the application of that science. Therefore, it celebrates management. The following chapter is drawn from the speech given by Melinda Gates to honor the first recipient of the award. This speech was first given on May 31, 2001, at the Global Health Council's Twenty-Eighth Annual Conference in Washington, D.C.

- Freedom from want

- Freedom from fear

These freedoms should not stop at any border, nor should they stop at the number four.

It is time to insist that freedom from easily preventable disease is a basic human right. A fifth freedom, more important than the others because it precedes them and makes them possible, we might call simply the "freedom to grow up."

The Gates Foundation was created in 1994. This is a short time by some measures. It is a lifetime by others. Most Americans, following the rise of the stock market, think these last years were years of unimpeded progress. It is true that in the developed world, new technology has changed peoples' lives forever. It certainly has changed mine! Thanks to computers, the Internet, biotechnology, and DNA research, we now think very differently about the basic organization of life. But whenever I hear about how great we are doing, I know that it is time for a reality check:

- Only about 7 percent of the world's population is online.

- Half the world's people have never made a phone call, much less sent a fax or an e-mail.

- Half live on less than $2 a day.

- They overwhelmingly lack sanitation and clean water.

- Almost a billion adults cannot read.

Although the "information age" has changed many of our lives, it has not changed most lives at all. And our new knowledge of life's inner workings has done too little to save lives in the developing world.

People often ask my husband and me why we decided to make global health the top priority of our foundation. Our decision is rooted in a belief all global health workers embody in their daily work: the loss of a child in one place on the planet is no less tragic than the loss of a child in another.

It is unacceptable that a plane crash is considered worldwide news, but the fact that fifty times as many people die of preventable diseases the same day, and every day, is never mentioned.

It is unacceptable that any child of the twenty-first century—let alone three million each year—dies because we fail to get them the vaccines they need. If we can make a difference, then we have to make a difference.

There is a nice quote used by the Global Health Council: "When it comes to global health, there is no 'them'; there is only us." The last decade has shown the many ways we connect with each other. We must never forget that connection brings responsibility.

I am reminded of something Nelson Mandela wrote to the people of South Africa in 1985, when he was still in jail on Robben Island: "Your freedom and mine cannot be separated."

It does not take a scientist to know that our health, like our freedom, is ultimately indivisible. I think all of us instinctively feel that. And more and more of us feel that freedom and human rights are only platitudes if we cannot do more to help people around the world attain a basic level of health that makes those values worth cherishing.

As Bill and I began to explore where we could make the greatest impact with our resources, we were stunned to learn how many lives are being saved—and how many more could be saved—by providing access to simple interventions such as vaccines.

Why should there be a fifteen-year lag between when a vaccine is available in the West and when it is available in developing countries? The answer is simple: there should not be. If a hepatitis B vaccine is available in the United States, it should be available everywhere.

When an AIDS [acquired immunodeficiency syndrome] vaccine is developed, it must be available everywhere. We have met a lot of health professionals since the foundation started, and nothing has inspired our commitment more than the work of global health workers on the front lines—those providing grassroots management. Day after day, year after year, they are leading the fight against disease and poverty, the most important job in the world.

I was deeply moved during a recent trip to India as I spoke with a young doctor at an AIDS hospice. This doctor told me how in this home, they virtually bring people back to life by "the simple act of treating them by our hearts."

The fight against AIDS is going to take all of our hearts and minds and political will—as well as a generous sharing of our resources. But we can, and we must, stop this terrible disease.

Secretary-General Annan has rightly said that AIDS is "the world's biggest public health challenge" and "in some countries, the biggest single obstacle to development." In Africa, what should have been a decade of liberation—Nelson Mandela's decade—was instead something far less euphoric. An entire generation has been lost to AIDS.

And the question before us today is whether a decade from now, we will have tens of millions or hundreds of millions infected. This is not merely an African problem. In the Caribbean, in Eastern Europe and Russia, and especially in India, there are signs that AIDS is spreading. And spreading on a massive scale.

Yes, certain countries have shown leadership, among them Uganda, Senegal, and Thailand. But no one should mistake a stalemate for a victory, especially when there is so much more we have to do with both treatment and prevention.

I am encouraged that the U.S. government is committed to this fight and that Secretary [Colin] Powell has emphasized that global health is essential to global stability.

I strongly support Secretary-General Annan's call to action and urge the U.S. government and other donor nations to commit unprecedented resources to the fight against AIDS. The world can stop AIDS, but only if wealthy countries, starting with the United States, increase spending on AIDS in a dramatic way.

The Gates Award for Global Health celebrates the lives, the work, and the daily management abilities of many unsung heroes. It brings overdue recognition to the heroic people and institutions that have been fighting this fight for so long.

The Gates Award for Global Health was created to provide a million dollars to an organization that has made a major and lasting contribution to global health. In the first year, nominations came in from every continent, for organizations large and small, new and old, famous and obscure.

The decision was difficult, as you can imagine. With the first award, we recognized how much good science happens on the front lines, and we celebrated an organization that has swiftly moved from one problem to another, helping sufferers and scientists with equal selflessness.

It was a thrill to present the first Gates Award for Global Health to the Center for Health and Population Research in Bangladesh. The center has been in existence since 1960. Many of you know it as ICDDR,B—the International Center for Diarrheal Disease Research, Bangladesh.

The center's most famous achievement was their pioneering work in the development and dissemination of oral rehydration solution (ORS), a balance of sodium and glucose that is estimated to save the lives of three million children each year. Until ORS, one of the greatest killers in Bangladesh and across the developing world was diarrhea.

Most Americans do not know that diarrhea was a terrible killer during our own history. Walt Whitman, who served as a nurse during the war, said the Civil War was "about ninety-nine parts diarrhea to one part glory" (Traubel, 1982).

The simplicity of ORS should never obscure its brilliance or its impact. The center has also been in the forefront of the fight against cholera. It has become an important resource for family planning and nutritional information. And, of course, they treat people: 120,000 a year, more than 300 a day, 80 percent of whom are under five.

In both the Dhaka hospital and in Matlab, hours away by land and water, children are brought in all day long more dead than alive. They often leave the same day, with a new lease on life. We may understand the science behind that, but it does not make it any less of a miracle.

Best of all, the center's remarkable trainees are drawn from around the world, and they take their lessons back to their countries. More than twenty thousand trainees have come from and returned to seventy-eight countries. Each is an emissary of hope.

The great Nobel laureate and poet Rabindranath Tagore (1971) once wrote a poem that goes to the heart of the center's work. It embodies what all of us are trying to do for the world's children:

> You have burst the bond of darkness
> You are tiny, but are not little
> For all the lights in the world are your kin

References

Tagore, R. "Glow-Worm," *Sheaves: Poems and Songs*. Selected and translated by N. Gupta. Westport, Conn.: Greenwood Press, 1971.

Traubel, H. *With Walt Whitman in Camden*. Carbondale, Ill.: Southern Illinois University Press, 1982.

2

A New Role for Corporate America

Partners in Global Health and Development

Raymond V. Gilmartin

Although globalization and free markets have lifted hundreds of millions of people out of poverty, progress still eludes hundreds of millions more. This is a concern not just for philosophers and humanitarians. Whether and how the world's poor gain access to the benefits of globalization will be a key factor in defining the political, business, and economic climates for companies such as Merck and Company, Inc., in coming years.

Corporations have traditionally been reluctant to engage with these issues. But just as transnational challenges affect private citizens and governments in a variety of ways, corporations, too, must wrestle with the uncertainties of this new world. We live in a time when severe acute respiratory syndrome (SARS) in China can send red ink flowing from Thai airlines to Toronto theaters. A civil war in Central Africa can hamper Asia's microchip production.

A limited view is no longer tenable. Corporations need workable long-term business models that contribute to progress in the global economy, not just because it may improve corporate reputation but—more importantly—because investing in growth simply makes good business sense. This means developing, within our long-term strategies and business plans, policies for following and responding to political, social, and economic developments. And it means transforming our corporate responsibility efforts into effective tools for addressing, in partnership with others, the social challenges that threaten economic growth.

I saw the full spectrum of Merck's corporate responsibility efforts firsthand during a recent trip to Africa where I visited the medical school at the University of Cape Town. Its dean, Dr. Nicky Paday-achee, had been able to finish medical school because of a scholar-ship from Merck. While I visited the school, Padayachee took me on a tour of the new wing of the Cape Town medical school library, which Merck helped fund. This is classic corporate philanthropy—where a company provides funding to support causes that are con-sistent with its business—in our case, medical education and a medical library.

I also visited Tanzania to help celebrate the fifteenth anniver-sary of the Merck Mectizan Donation Program. There I had the opportunity to deliver the 250 millionth free dose of Mectizan (iver-mectin) to a woman in a small village, Bombani. The Mectizan Donation Program demonstrates a second—and deeper—level of corporate engagement (Sturchio and Colatrella, 2002). In the mid-1980s, Merck made the decision to donate Mectizan—a once-a-year treatment for river blindness—for as long as needed to as many peo-ple who need it. Today, river blindness is nearly vanquished.

I also traveled to Botswana, where, along with President Festus Mogae, I visited the village of Palapye, where we broke ground for a center for AIDS (acquired immunodeficiency syndrome) orphans called the House of Hope. We also visited Serowe and opened an AIDS treatment and counseling center.

That country, which is roughly the size of Texas, has a popula-tion of 1.7 million people, and more than a third of its citizens—37 percent of the entire adult population—are infected with the human immunodeficiency virus (HIV). In Botswana, Merck has taken corporate involvement in global health to an even more ambitious level. Through a partnership with the government and the Bill and Melinda Gates Foundation, we have created a truly comprehensive program to address HIV/AIDS (Distlerath and Mac-donald, 2004). This kind of partnership—among a pharmaceutical company, a foundation, and a nation-state—is extraordinary. We are seeking to create a model that other countries and companies can follow to conquer HIV/AIDS.

Our efforts in Africa demonstrate three important principles:

- First, improving global health is not merely a charitable goal: it is a business imperative.

- Second, global health care issues, such as HIV/AIDS, must be addressed in a comprehensive way.

- Third, no one company—or even one country—can address global health challenges alone. Complex health care problems require partnerships and collaborations to really engage and solve problems.

Improving Global Health Is a Business Imperative

Global health—and the grinding poverty that often leads to ill health—is a defining issue of our time. For corporations to maintain and extend markets from the developed world to emerging markets and on to all the nations of the world, we must create a foundation of political and economic stability that can only come by addressing global health challenges.

Corporations must view these issues from the perspective of a long-term investor. Addressing global health will help shape the political, business, and economic environments in which companies such as Merck will operate. It will shape an environment that leads to greater economic growth. It will shape a world that supports and defends a global trading partnership that promotes prosperity in poor nations and rich nations alike.

Whereas philanthropy remains an important role for corporate America, finding workable, long-term business models is the only real path to sustaining corporate involvement in fighting global health challenges such as AIDS, malaria, and tuberculosis. The World Bank has suggested, for example, that Africa's per capita growth rate from

1990 to 1997 would have been almost three times as high without the effects of HIV/AIDS. In sub-Saharan Africa, malaria is thought to shave half a point off economic growth rates every year. On the other hand, effective health policy has been a critical foundation for growth in developing countries. A recent Harvard study suggests a 0.3 percent increase in gross domestic product for every 10 percent reduction in malaria incidence (Gallup and Sachs, 2001).

As Merck and other global corporations look ahead, we see our best prospects for growth in the same emerging economies identified as the next generation of possible AIDS catastrophes—including China, India, and Russia. In too many of these countries, health care systems are inadequate to meet the crisis, and government responses have been too slow. Failure to act will devastate the employee base, the customer base, and the national economies that support business—not in ten to twenty years but in three to five years.

In India, experts now say that the epidemic is following the same arc as Africa's in the 1980s, with the potential for similar rates of infection. Two University of California scientists have predicted that as many as twenty-five million people in India may be HIV-positive by 2010 (Gordon, 2002). Treating just 10 percent of them with low-cost domestic drugs would cost on the order of $900 million annually—three times India's national health budget and one-third the government's annual expenditure on research and development. Such expenditures would clearly be unsustainable. China, Russia, Ukraine, Nigeria, South Africa, Indonesia—all potential engines for regional and global growth—face similar threats.

Prescription for Success

Comprehensive Programs, Strong Partnerships

Global disease is both a cause and an effect of poverty. As we learned in Botswana, beginning to deal with disease and its effects involves building the necessary human and physical infrastructure of health care. It means training physicians and nurses; it means building hospitals, treatment centers, and testing facilities; it means providing teacher training and basic education in schools; and sadly, it means recognizing that we have to attend to a generation of orphans on whose future a nation depends.

Developing these comprehensive approaches is difficult, complex, costly, and time consuming. Tackling global health changes requires partnerships and collaborations. I suggest that corporations have an opportunity to play a significant role, and a much broader role, than the private sector has traditionally played in creating and participating in partnerships for global health and development.

Our experiences have taught us that any successful partnership in global health begins with the following six factors in place.

Take Time to Study What Is Needed

Fully understand the challenges involved. Our first effort to help launch a workplace HIV/AIDS program with customers in South Africa, for example, was disappointing because we had not anticipated the extent to which fear and stigma would prevent workers from signaling their HIV status on the job. The reason: workers were suspicious, thinking they would face discrimination or be fired if they admitted being HIV-positive. This taught us that HIV is as much a social as a medical phenomenon, and solutions must fit within communities, not stand apart from them.

Assemble a Broad Range of Partners

It is tempting—and sounds efficient—to go it alone. But our experience with river blindness showed that it was critical to work closely with nongovernmental organizations (NGOs) that were already delivering care to remote villages and with government health officials to ensure that the Mectizan Donation Program was effectively integrated with the national health system. We learned similar lessons in Botswana, where the multisectoral approach coordinated by the government has mobilized community groups, faith-based organizations, and other sectors of civil society to help in the fight against HIV/AIDS. These experiences have led us to believe that involving more partners, bringing local ownership and expertise, makes success more likely.

Agree on a Shared Set of Goals

Successful collaboration is based on common objectives, mutual respect, and benefits for all the partners involved. Starting with a clear set of feasible targets and monitoring progress regularly are two important success factors. For example, the Merck-Gates project in Botswana began with a formal agreement with the government outlining a governance structure, shared goals, and agreement on responsibilities, decision making, and reporting processes. The work of the partnership is firmly integrated with the national comprehensive HIV/AIDS strategy.

Secure High-Level Commitment and Engagement

Without political will on the part of national leadership, success is unlikely. This is clear from global experience with the HIV epidemic: the countries that have made significant progress—Botswana, Brazil, Senegal, Thailand, and Uganda—could count on the unequivocal commitment of senior political leaders. At the same time, partners are right to seek high-level corporate participation as a sign of seriousness and staying power. We have been told that the participation of senior Merck executives made us a more attractive partner, and we also look for high-level involvement when we choose partners.

Focus on the Long Term

Projects must be sustainable for the recipients, which means integrating them with local health systems and empowering local officials wherever possible. But they must also be sustainable for corporations, particularly where medicines are concerned, lest programs end by worsening the condition they were intended to treat.

This means that corporations must make a long-term commitment and have the sound financial base to live up to it. This is precisely what Merck has done in Botswana and also in the Mectizan Donation Program (now in its seventeenth year).

Recognize the Need for Transparency

Making progress in global health is difficult and complex. Cynicism and suspicion are to be expected. But rather than ignore reasonable concerns, successful public-private partnerships address them openly. The Mectizan Donation Program, for instance, is administered by an independent expert committee that regularly reviews program policies and achievements. And, as noted above, the collaboration in Botswana is fully integrated with the government response to HIV/AIDS, with regular reviews with relevant public- and private-sector partners. Transparency and tangible accomplishments that bring new resources and health improvement to affected communities will ultimately be the best way to build trust and confidence among stakeholders.

Two Decades of Lessons Learned

Like everyone who has worked in international development, we have learned many lessons over the years, and the learning process has taken us places we never imagined. Our Mectizan Donation Program, conceived twenty years ago as a drug donation initiative, turned into a partnership involving dozens of countries and entities, two diseases, and a range of health infrastructure concerns. Similarly, we see our AIDS initiatives evolving from public concern over the price of medicines to coalitions delivering not just drugs but also training, education, and infrastructure. Other corporations report similar experiences. The potential for philanthropic "mission creep" is unnerving. But rather than turn away, we and others are finding it possible to meet the challenge.

More than two decades ago, Merck developed a simple, safe, and effective once-a-year treatment for river blindness (onchocerciasis) that had the potential to prevent millions of people in some of the poorest countries in the world from losing their sight and, with it, the ability to support a family.

At first, our doubts that donating the drug would be the right course of action were matched by health community doubts that we had the right drug or the right approach. Yet, building ties with the World Health Organization (WHO) and making the internal decision to donate the drug for as long as needed wherever needed turned out to be relatively easy compared with the challenges of getting it to patients. We had little or no presence in the countries most heavily affected; many of them had limited health infrastructure in the areas we needed to reach. We found that meeting our commitment to provide the drug meant taking the lead in assembling a coalition to get it to those in need.

By 2002, after fifteen years, an unprecedented public-private partnership—including the Carter Center; aid agencies; international organizations like WHO, the United Nations Children's Fund (UNICEF), and the World Bank; national ministries of health; and dozens of nongovernmental groups—was providing Mectizan to more than thirty million people each year in thirty-three of the thirty-five nations where the disease is endemic. Infection rates in some places have fallen from 50 percent to close to zero; farmers in affected areas have returned to fertile land.

The whole project could have failed if we had rushed ahead before we understood the challenges of delivering so simple a product. It almost did fail when we sought to manage Mectizan with roaming mobile teams—not a feasible approach for covering thirty-three countries over fifteen years. Experience has proved that experts could train communities to direct and manage their own treatment—with minimal outside involvement after an initial five years. Now more than sixty-one thousand communities conduct their own treatment programs—testimony to the power of local ownership and involvement.

What had been conceived as a drug donation program evolved into a broad public health initiative implemented through a pioneering public-private partnership. With Mectizan, we began to understand that to make philanthropic resources more effective, or even to make them effective at all, they had to be used more strategically in partnerships that had broader impact on health care delivery in affected countries. Some had feared that the Mectizan Donation Program would discourage research into diseases of the poor. Yet, once our public-private partnership began to function well and grow, it had the opposite effect. Recently, GlaxoSmithKline, Inc., joined the coalition with its treatment for the tropical disease lymphatic filariasis, benefiting from the already established distribution structure, and Merck extended our program to donate Mectizan for the treatment of this disease in countries where it is coendemic with river blindness. The initiative also served as a model for the International Trachoma Initiative, which brings together Pfizer, the Edna McConnell Clark Foundation, and WHO.

Responding to HIV/AIDS

As did many global firms, Merck found in recent years that responding to the HIV/AIDS pandemic was not an option but a strategic and humanitarian necessity. We drew two lessons from our Mectizan experience: first, that discounted medicines alone were not the solution; and second, that we did not know enough to say what the solution was for the developing world, let alone put it into practice.

Our work on HIV/AIDS issues began with a broad HIV/AIDS research program, which led to the discovery of two antiretroviral medicines, Crixivan (indinivir sulfate) and Stocrin (efavirenz). This program continues today with our efforts to find a safe and effective HIV vaccine and our research on an integrase inhibitor. Our work in the HIV/AIDS arena expanded when we provided a grant to establish the Enhancing Care Initiative at the Harvard AIDS Institute and the Francois-Xavier Bagnoud Center at the Harvard School of

Public Health. The enhancing care initiative supported in-country teams in Brazil, Thailand, Senegal, and KwaZulu Natal in South Africa, and in Puerto Rico, to assess local needs, develop strategies to address HIV/AIDS, and work to promote change at the country level.

In 2000, we joined four other research-based pharmaceutical companies (Boehringer-Ingelheim, Bristol-Myers Squibb, F. Hoffmann-La Roche, and GlaxoSmithKline) and five United Nations agencies (the Joint United Nations Program for HIV/AIDS [UNAIDS], WHO, UNICEF, the U.N. Population Fund, and the World Bank) in the Accelerating Access Initiative aimed at both reducing drug prices and building relationships with developing countries that were committed to strengthening national responses to the HIV/AIDS epidemic. This collaboration between the public and private sectors was unprecedented, but those involved were frustrated by the relatively slow pace at which additional patients gained access to treatment. To catalyze further action, Merck announced its decision to sell our two current HIV/AIDS medicines at prices at which we would not profit in some sixty of the least-developed countries and those hardest hit by AIDS and at significantly reduced prices in nearly sixty additional countries.

By December 2003, through the efforts of Accelerating Access Initiative companies (later joined by Abbott Laboratories and Gilead), more than 150,000 additional people in sub-Saharan Africa gained access to antiretroviral therapy. The number of patients with access to therapy doubled in the last six months of 2003—an encouraging sign—and the quality of the treatment had increased (as indicated by the percentage of patients receiving triple combination therapy). For the two Merck drugs involved, this represented a sixteenfold increase in less than three years, but the drugs were still reaching only a small fraction of those in need. Rates of infection were still increasing in all but a few places, and societies were increasingly showing the strains.

Something more was urgently needed: a comprehensive approach in which communities gained improved access to treatment and also prevention, care, and infrastructure support. Drug providers would have to partner with government and private organizations, each offering their particular resources and expertise and taking responsibility for a share of the solution. With this learning in mind, we set out to build a public-private initiative that would provide a comprehensive response to HIV/AIDS in one country.

No step along this road has been easy. Initially, many foundations and NGOs were deeply suspicious of our motives and commitment. After much discussion, our visible high-level commitment and previous record helped convince the Bill and Melinda Gates Foundation to work with us. Our common concept—comprehensive support for the HIV/AIDS program of one committed national government—proved attractive to other partners, such as the Centers for Disease Control and Prevention and the Harvard AIDS Institute. In large part because of the outstanding leadership of President Festus Mogae, the government of Botswana became our African country partner in what was named the African Comprehensive HIV/AIDS Partnerships.

We were determined from the outset that this model would be fully integrated with Botswana's national AIDS strategy. That meant that for the project's first six months, the outside partners provided resources and expertise to help Botswana draw up its plan.

We also recognized that limitations in human resources and infrastructure created major barriers to progress, so we focused on training health care workers; passing on managerial and technical skills; and developing education, marketing, and health services that citizens of Botswana would be able to sustain and share. We had not expected to find ourselves so involved in building not just medical but also leadership skills. But we have been told that our abilities in this area—something for which private business is uniquely suited—are perhaps the most vital quality we bring to the partnership.

The Merck Company Foundation and the Bill and Melinda Gates Foundation each will provide U.S.$50 million over the next five years to fund these initiatives and also AIDS prevention, condom distribution, treatment, and family support. Merck is also donating antiretroviral drugs for the duration of the partnership.

Early results are encouraging, and the Botswana project is picking up momentum. Training programs on HIV/AIDS care and antiretroviral therapy are now available to every health care professional in Botswana; more than twenty-seven thousand people are enrolled in the national AIDS treatment program, and more than seventeen thousand are already receiving antiretroviral drugs (as of June 2004). We are still learning and working to expand our range of local partners to mobilize Botswana's private sector and to involve traditional healers. Although Botswana's experience is unique, we expect the model—built on close collaboration between the public and private sectors and a comprehensive approach to the national response—to offer important lessons that can be adapted to other countries heavily affected by HIV/AIDS.

At the same time, we are learning from the experiences of other corporations, motivated both by internal pressures—the increasing toll of health issues, in particular, on corporate prospects in the developing world—and by external calls from nongovernmental groups and other stakeholders for more corporate response. Smart companies, instead of resisting, are working to see how the demands of the bottom line and good citizenship can be harnessed to the same plow:

- DaimlerChrysler has been widely recognized for its workplace AIDS program in South Africa, working with trade unions, the government, and GTZ, a German aid agency, to implement workplace education, testing, and counseling for, and treatment of, HIV/AIDS. When the program began in 2000, it focused only on ameliorating the toll AIDS took on employee health and productivity. But a more thorough understanding of the effects of AIDS on the company emerged as the issue was studied, and now the company's core goal has broadened into "secur[ing] the sustainability of its investment and operations in the country." Next steps for this program include sharing education, training, and DaimlerChrysler health services with local communities and South African government entities such as the National Tuberculosis Control Program (Seitz, Staber, and Jonczyk, 2002).

- The Coca-Cola Company has faced a similar blend of unrelenting public pressure to do more on AIDS and in-house questions about the viability of African markets where 15 to 35 percent of its young customer group is dying of the disease. It established a corporate foundation, the Coca-Cola Africa Foundation, that manages support for AIDS prevention and education across Africa. In 2001, those programs expanded into partnership with UNAIDS, with Coca-Cola pledging to use its distribution network and marketing capabilities to support local education, prevention, and treatment programs and to "develop and implement model human resources policies and practices" for its employees. Most recently, the foundation joined forces with two NGOs, pharmaceutical firms, and forty African bottling companies to offer the bottlers' employees expanded health care benefits, including access to antiretroviral drugs (Global Business Coalition on HIV/AIDS, 2005).

Each of these examples started out as responses to problems with the bottom line—spiraling health costs and, in at least one case, mounting public criticism. But, as Karl-Heinz Schlaiss of Daimler-Chrysler has remarked, an initial focus on workplace problems gave way to an understanding that the effect of disease on society, and on long-term business prospects, required a much broader response.

Corporations, governments, and NGOs are beginning to recognize that a continued narrow focus on each institution's internal goals is no longer sufficient to meet the expectations others set of us—or the goals that we have set for ourselves.

There is more to do to make public-private partnerships better understood and accepted. Leaders from government, international organizations, and NGOs need to think about how they can encourage corporate involvement to meet global needs. Today, outsiders often perceive multinational corporations as more powerful than they actually are; this gives rise to the temptation to turn to us, as one analyst has put it, as a "default key" when national, international, and civic institutions have failed (Freeman, 2002).

This is not the right approach. Government, civil society, and the international community must bear the primary responsibility for meeting citizens' basic needs—and mediating relations with the market and its corporate citizens. Corporations are ill suited to supply the basic building blocks of governance—and, when asked to do so, have not often succeeded.

Whereas governments and NGOs do themselves a service by understanding what corporations are suited to do, corporations should recognize that dealing with NGOs and other actors in civil society is an integral part of their role. BP's chief executive Lord John Browne (2002) has said, "It is a mistake sometimes reflected in media coverage to think that companies and NGOs are locked into an immutably hostile relationship. That isn't true. Companies benefit from scrutiny and challenge, and in some of the most complex areas in which we work, the progress we can make is dependent on the cooperation and skills of NGOs."

A host of initiatives—from trade groups to geographical groupings such as the Corporate Council on Africa, the Global Health Council to the Global Business Coalition on HIV/AIDS, or the World Economic Forum's Global Health Initiative—offer companies the opportunity to learn from what others are doing. And government agencies (like USAID and its counterparts in the United Kingdom and Germany) and international organizations (through such initiatives as the United Nation's Global Compact or the bilateral efforts of the World Bank, UNICEF, WHO, and other agencies) are also reaching out to encourage corporate engagement in global health issues.

The future will offer more challenges like HIV/AIDS: the search for vaccines for malaria, tuberculosis, rotavirus, and cervical cancer; the costly challenge of the diseases of aging in rich and poor societies alike; and the growing gap between expectations and resources confronting health care systems all over the world. For Merck, some of these health challenges represent professional opportunities, but for us and for every global company, understanding and responding effectively to the tangle of economic, environmental, and security problems that surround health are keys to future growth.

Today we have the possibility of sharing benefits that corporate leaders might not have imagined fifty years ago. But we cannot do it without partners who share our belief that if we can find the right way to work together, drawing on the ingenuity and commitment of all stakeholders, with corporations working side by side with their partners in civil society and in government alike, the right results will follow.

References

Browne, Lord John. Speech on "International Relations: The New Agenda for Business," Feb. 27, 2002, Chatham House, London.

Distlerath, L. M., and Macdonald, G. "The African Comprehensive HIV/AIDS Partnerships—A New Role for Multinational Companies in Global Health Policy." *Yale Journal of Health Policy, Law and Ethics*, 2004, 4(1), 147–155.

Freeman, B. "Responsible Companies." *Johannesburg Summit 2002—Challenges and Partnerships*, Official UN Division for Sustainable Development WWSD [World Summit on Sustainable Development] Publication. Feb. 8, 2002. Available: http://www.iblf.org/csr/csrwebassist.nsf/550d4b 46b29f68a6852568660081f938/80256adc002b820480256c3e00578deb/ $FILE/pp48-50(freeman).pdf. Accessed: Jan. 5, 2005.

Gallup, J. L., and Sachs, J. D. "The Economic Burden of Malaria." *American Journal of Tropical Medicine and Hygiene*, Jan. 2001, 64, 85–96.

Global Business Coalition on HIV/AIDS. "HIV/AIDS Program Description." Available: www.businessfightsaids.org/site/apps/nl/content2.asp?c= nmK0LaP6E&b=239558&ct=283052. Accessed: Jan. 5, 2005.

Gordon, D. F. "The Next Wave of HIV/AIDS: Nigeria, Ethiopia, Russia, India, and China." *Intelligence Community Assessment,* National Intelligence Council, Sept. 2002. Available: http://www.odci.gov/nic/special_ nextwaveHIV.html. Accessed: January 4, 2005.

"Mectizan Compendium." *Tropical Medicine and International Health,* 2004, 9(3), A1–A56.

Seitz, B., Staber, U., and Jonczyk, C. "Case Study: DaimlerChrysler South Africa—Dealing with the Effects of HIV/AIDS on Human and Social Capital," UN Global Compact Learning Forum, Dec. 2, 2002. Available: www.unglobalcompact.org/Portal/. Accessed: Jan. 5, 2005.

Sturchio, J. L., and Colatrella, B. D. "Successful Public-Private Partnerships in Global Health: Lessons from the Mectizan Donation Program." In B. Granville (ed.), *Economics of Essential Medicines.* London: Royal Institute of International Affairs, 2002, pp. 255–274.

3

From Challenges to Policy

Lee Jong-wook

Health hazards have always been present, but they have not always been as keenly felt as they are now. "The euphoria of the age of penicillin or the 'pill' has turned to anxiety," remarked Roy Porter in 1997 (p. 716). He cited alarms about cholera, plague, and cloned humans. We could add severe acute respiratory syndrome, Creutzfeldt-Jakob disease, Ebola virus, avian influenza, anthrax, smallpox, acquired immunodeficiency syndrome (AIDS), tuberculosis, malaria, cancer, obesity, and other dangers, old and new, including an expanding array of natural or human-caused catastrophes.

In the early days of the World Health Organization (WHO), by contrast, a prevalent view was that science and technology were now strong enough to solve most of the world's health problems. As Brock Chisholm, the first director-general of WHO from 1948 to 1953, reminisced (1995, p. 393): "The microbe was no longer the main enemy: science was sufficiently advanced to be able to cope with it admirably, if it were not for such barriers as superstition, ignorance, religious intolerance, misery, and poverty."

Chisholm supported mass campaigns against tuberculosis and smallpox by vaccination, malaria mainly by spraying DDT, and yaws by administering penicillin. Yaws control met with rapid success, and smallpox was eventually eradicated. But malaria and tuberculosis control ran into difficulties, arguably because they were never conducted on a big-enough scale to make the decisive difference needed. Underestimating the resources needed had been a difficulty from the start. In 1951, V. Nalliah, the delegate from Ceylon (now Sri Lanka), told the World Health Assembly:

"The Director-General of WHO is today finding it difficult to collect together a paltry eight million dollars. . . . We are also reminded that there are nations which are prepared to spend 60 billion dollars on defense. I say that the surest way to bring peace into the world is to encourage activities of organizations of this nature." (*World Health Forum*, 1998, p. 24).

Already for the previous biennium, the budget adopted in 1949 had been U.S.$5 million instead of the U.S.$6.5 million to U.S.$7 million recommended by the Interim Commission on the basis of the program it had "carefully and cautiously prepared." Karl Evang, the delegate from Norway to the World Health Assembly, criticized this decision bitterly:

"I am not surprised at the lack of imagination and vision expressed in this drastic cut. . . . What to my mind is surprising is the lack of realism and of practical sense of which this decision carries proof. We are public health people, not representatives of treasury departments. We know that action is needed, and we know that we cannot convince anybody unless we take action. To take action, you have to be an operating agency—to go out into the field and do the work" (*World Health Forum*, 1998, p. 23).

The prospects for malaria eradication waned in many parts of the world with the need to discontinue DDT spraying owing to its toxic effects on the environment, and gradually talk of eradication was dropped altogether. Tuberculosis began its steady comeback, accelerated first by the rise of drug resistance, then by coinfection with HIV.

By the end of the 1980s, the behavior both of pathogens and of human beings had turned out to be less tractable than expected. First defined in 1982, AIDS was spreading rapidly worldwide, with health education and condoms as the only means of preventing sexual transmission, and no means of treatment. The number of deaths from tuberculosis and malaria continued to rise, despite the existence of effective tools for treatment and prevention. These three diseases, fueled by poverty and fueling more poverty in their turn, were seen as a major global threat to health at the end of the twentieth century.

"Combat HIV/AIDS, malaria, and other diseases" was made one of eight Millennium Development Goals adopted by the global community with a United Nations declaration in 2000. To attract and disburse the funding needed to control these three diseases, the Group of Eight (G8) countries (Canada, France, Germany, Italy, Japan, Russia, United Kingdom, and United States), the United Nations, and the World Bank set up the Global Fund to Fight AIDS, Tuberculosis and Malaria, which went into operation in 2002 and was supporting 225 programs worth U.S.$2.1 billion by March 2004 (Nebehay, 2004). Development assistance for health through bilateral and other donors has been increasing during the past three years. These beginnings of a mobilization against today's main disease threat are welcome, but for them to succeed, specific strategies have to be worked out in detail and pursued with determination within the context of broad support for health sector development.

To attack on all fronts at once and with equal force is no more possible in the struggle for health than in any other kind of struggle. It is probably even less possible in public health than elsewhere because the demand for reduced illness and postponed death is probably infinite, whereas the supply of means for meeting it is certainly finite. An objective has to be chosen that embodies the main problem and is both ambitious enough to mobilize maximum effort and realistic enough to be achievable.

A Twenty-First-Century Initiative

The availability of a treatment that stops the progression of AIDS within the human body brings the long-hoped-for opportunity to make inroads into the HIV (human immunodeficiency virus)/AIDS pandemic. Antiretroviral therapy can restore patients to normal life for an as-yet-unknown amount of time and can therefore halt the destruction HIV/AIDS is currently causing in the lives of individuals, families, communities, and whole societies.

HIV/AIDS has killed more than thirty million people and is the most devastating disease the world has faced for several centuries. In Africa, transmission of HIV has been accelerated by poverty, gender inequality, and health systems weakened by external debt. More than 70 percent of those infected with HIV now live on that continent, and most AIDS deaths have occurred there. The spread of HIV has reversed gains in life expectancy in many of these countries and orphaned an estimated fourteen million children. A recent World Bank study predicted that South Africa would face "complete economic collapse . . . within three generations" (World Health Organization, 2003b) if that country did not take effective measures to combat AIDS.

In the 1980s and early 1990s, North America, Europe, Australia, and Japan had been faced with the same danger but were able to mobilize enough resources for public information, education, condoms, and blood safety to contain it. Antiretroviral treatment came into use in these countries later in the 1990s and, despite the high cost, was quickly made accessible to many of those who needed it. Since then, the death rates from HIV/AIDS have dropped in rich countries but have continued to rise in poor ones.

By the end of 2003, there were an estimated forty million people living with HIV/AIDS (World Health Organization, 2003b). Six million of them will die during the next two years unless they obtain treatment. At present, poverty prevents them from doing so. Most of those six million are surviving in communities that are already severely weakened by AIDS illness and deaths. Those who do obtain treatment normally recover health and are able to go back to work, look after their families, and participate in building a society that can protect itself against disease and malnutrition. There can be no question about whether they should receive treatment, only about how much time is needed to get it to them. The facilities to produce the drugs in the quantities needed and at affordable prices are still under construction. Time is also needed to train a large enough number of health workers in the necessary diagnosis and treatment procedures, equip and organize the health services, and set up the necessary procurement and distribution services.

The origin of the much-discussed "3-by-5" initiative is a meeting of the Joint United Nations Program for HIV/AIDS (UNAIDS) held in 2001, in which the participants designed a best-case scenario whereby three million people in developing countries would be receiving antiretroviral therapy by the end of 2005 (Schwartlander and others, 2001). The numerical target expresses the challenge in the simplest and yet most demanding terms possible. It is ambitious in that it would require every organization involved in HIV/AIDS control to work to its maximum capacity, but that is what they want to do anyway. Once the challenge had been formulated, the logic behind it and the possibility it represents became inescapable.

WHO responded by committing itself to doing everything it can within its mandate and resources to achieve this target: normative work at a pace never before seen in HIV control, a rapid expansion of technical support to countries, convening of partners to coordinate their efforts, and global advocacy to maximize political and material support. As with any ambitious project, many have questioned its feasibility and argue that a lower number or a later year would have been better. These arguments are of interest but only to the extent that they help to define the obstacles. As we find out what they are, we can work through them one by one until we reach our objective: universal access to treatment. The questions about how to get there are a matter not of academic debate but of specific and practical engineering.

It is certainly not something that one agency can achieve on its own. Indispensable for such an undertaking is close working relations and alliances that combine the necessary expertise and resources. We are working in four equally important kinds of partnership.

First is the partnership of WHO with international organizations, particularly UNAIDS, which combines and coordinates resources from nine U.N. organizations (United Nations Children's Fund [UNICEF], World Food Program, United Nations Development Program, United Nations Population Fund, United Nations Office on Drugs and Crime, International Labor Organization, United Nations Educational, Scientific and Cultural Organization [UNESCO], WHO, and the World Bank); and the Global Fund, which is also a partnership, in its own words, "between governments, civil society, the private sector, and affected communities to channel funds for the control of HIV/AIDS, tuberculosis, and malaria" (http://www.theglobalfund.org). Around this core of three organizations are the many other international agencies we are working with regarding particular aspects of the initiative, such as UNICEF on protecting children from infection, UNESCO on health education, and the Office of the United Nations High Commissioner for Human Rights on equitable access to treatment.

Next, between the global and local levels, is the partnership between these agencies and their public- and private-sector donors. These include bilateral aid, support from foundations, and work with suppliers to obtain equipment and supplies on the most favorable terms possible. Donors in many cases opt for meeting particular needs, such as medicines, facilities, or training programs. The AIDS Medicines and Diagnostics Service assists countries with purchasing drugs and diagnostics while working closely with the suppliers to keep them informed of demand, negotiate prices, and help coordinate regulatory procedures.

Then comes WHO's partnership with national and local health authorities. It is only by working with them that the international community can help to build up sustainable systems for the delivery of treatment and care. Existing services must be fully used, strengthened, and coordinated with prevention activities to take as much advantage as possible of the opportunities that treatment brings. Availability of treatment can increase the use of testing and counseling services by reducing stigma and the fear of death. Where more people use these services, the rate of HIV transmission declines.

This is where the fourth and equally indispensable kind of partnership comes in, with nongovernmental and community organizations. Some of the most effective HIV/AIDS prevention and control work in the world is being carried out by groups in this category. In many cases, better funding and technical support can enable them to replicate small projects and accelerate progress toward reaching the necessary scale of action. However, there is also a wide spectrum of opinions and commitments at this level of engagement, and harmonization requires determination, creativity, and courage.

Community participation can also be seen as a partnership, and the need and the potential for it is as great now as it was at the time of the Alma-Ata Declaration that launched the health-for-all movement in 1978. Community participation was defined then as "the process by which individuals assume responsibility for their own health and welfare and for those of the community." It was advocated because it enables people "to become agents of their own development instead of passive beneficiaries of development aid" (World Health Organization, 1978). A situation was envisaged in which health workers themselves were part of the community and could thus make full use of its existing organization and communication systems, to both understand health needs and make them better understood. In the case of HIV/AIDS control, this kind of knowledge and participation can be the key to essential activities: counseling and testing, support for safe practices, adherence to treatment, and provision of care. Where individuals and local groups are aware of a health need and have the means at their disposal of meeting it, a great deal is achieved even where resources are short.

Although specific major initiatives are probably always necessary, they must not be allowed to deprive other health programs of essential resources and energy. The idea of the 3-by-5 initiative is to do the opposite, by making one major effort act as a catalyst for others. The systems now being set up to provide lifelong care for people living with HIV/AIDS include training for nurses and community health workers; drug-quality monitoring for safety and efficacy; drug production, procurement, and distribution; surveillance, diagnosis, and treatment of HIV/AIDS, tuberculosis, and other opportunistic infections; public information and education for health; and counseling and testing services. Where these services are available, they can have multiple uses, and health systems are the stronger for them. They will contribute more and more to the control of other infectious and chronic diseases as the procedures for HIV/AIDS diagnosis and treatment become established.

A second contribution that intense emergency activity can make, potentially more beneficial still in the long run, is to catalyze new ideas about how to organize and finance health services. The epidemiological and social situation in every country is changing so rapidly that new approaches in this area are as urgently needed as new drugs and technologies for specific health problems.

Action as a Source of Ideas

A recent example in public health of action that generates creativity is the smallpox eradication campaign of the 1970s, which led to the Expanded Programme on Immunization and the health-for-all movement of the 1980s. More far-reaching, and perhaps more useful as a reference point for the kind of new thinking needed now, are some of the ideas that arose during and immediately after the Second World War.

In London in 1942, William Beveridge introduced to Parliament his report "Social Insurance and Allied Services" by observing: "The first principle is that any proposals for the future, while they should use to the full the experience gathered in the past, should not be restricted by consideration of sectional interests established in the obtaining of that experience. Now, when the war is abolishing landmarks of every kind, is the opportunity for using experience in a clear field. A revolutionary moment in the world's history is a time for revolutions, not for patching" (reprinted in 1955, pp. 845–846).

The U.K.'s National Health Service came into existence in 1946 on the basis of the recommendations Beveridge made in this report. Its emphasis was on universal coverage for every member of society, without distinction. In the expression WHO began to use in the 1970s, it was a practical financial model for "health for all," understood as access for all to an adequate minimum of health services. The establishment of universal, publicly financed health insurance was successful in the United Kingdom for several decades and admired and imitated by other countries. It was not fundamentally altered until 1989, when market-based reforms made general practitioners into fund holders and public money payable to private providers, but even now it survives to a debatable extent (Musgrove, 2000).

The Charter of the United Nations, signed on June 26, 1945, in San Francisco, was also catalyzed to a large extent by the devastation caused by the destruction of systems of justice and peace: "to save succeeding generations from the scourge of war, which twice in our lifetime has brought untold sorrow to mankind." Contrary to the expectations of many, and despite the unprecedented dangers the cold war represented, there were widespread increases in prosperity during the second half of the twentieth century. The rules and principles for peaceful coexistence set out in the charter cannot claim all the credit for these improvements, but it would be perverse to deny that they played an important part in them, if only by giving some idea of what would be desirable.

WHO's constitution, adopted in New York on July 22, 1946, sets out nine principles that are "basic to the happiness, harmonious relations, and security of all peoples." The first three define health as "a state of complete physical, mental, and social well-being"; assert that the enjoyment of the highest attainable standard of it is "one of the fundamental rights of every human being without distinction of race, religion, political belief, economic or social condition," and call for the "fullest co-operation of individuals and

States" in ensuring "the health of all peoples" because it is "funda-mental to the attainment of peace and security" (World Health Organization, 2003a). The other six are about how the governments of member states must help one another take the measures neces-sary to protect the health of their respective populations.

It is hard to imagine higher claims for health or a stronger com-mitment to making it as available as possible to everyone. As in the case of the U.N. charter, things turned out in some ways better than expected. By the end of the twentieth century, infant mortality had fallen from 156 per 1,000 live births in 1945 to 54 per 1,000; aver-age life expectancy had increased from forty-six to sixty-six years; smallpox had been eradicated; polio was approaching eradication; and the prospects were good for eliminating leprosy, measles, neona-tal tetanus, and micronutrient deficiencies. Economic and social factors have played a large part in achieving improvements of this kind, but so have international cooperation in health and the clear commitments that have inspired and guided it.

WHO came into existence with the twenty-sixth ratification of its constitution, in 1948. The year before, Albert Camus had pub-lished *The Plague*, the landmark novel that won him the Nobel prize. It describes the experience of a plague-stricken town, as observed by a physician. The narrator concludes that he wrote his account "to bear witness to the injustice and violence that had been done" to the people of that town "and simply to say what one learns during plagues, that there is more to admire in human beings than to despise" (p. 279). The plague is used as an analogy for a time of war, and he says, his account tells about "what had to be done and, doubtless, would have to be done again against terror and its relent-less armory, in spite of personal anguish, by everyone who, not being able to be saints and refusing to accept plagues, try nevertheless to be doctors" (p. 279).

Despite the many dangers of the 1940s and the abolition of landmarks referred to by Beveridge (1942), it was a time of unusual creativity, and the need for health played a central part. The kinds of dangers and challenges mentioned at the beginning of this chapter give some idea of the need for similar levels of creativity now. The 3-by-5 initiative can be seen as an early attempt to catalyze this kind of thinking. It seems evident that only a highly innovative and ambitious agenda of this kind is likely to steer us toward an acceptable future. If there is to be a viable level of justice and security in the world, the work of defining health and designing a framework for protecting and promoting it must be continued and renewed.

References

Beveridge, W. *Social Insurance and Allied Services*. London: Her Majesty's Stationery Office, 1942 [reprinted 1955].

Camus, A. *La Peste*. Paris: Gallimard, 1947.

Chisholm, B. "Words of Wisdom from the Past." *World Health Forum*, 1995, *16*(393), 70–73.

Musgrove, P. "Health Insurance: The Influence of the Beveridge Report." *Bulletin of the World Health Organization*, 2000, *78*, 845–846.

Nebehay, N. "Global Fund to Fight AIDS, Malaria, TB Faces Crunch." *Reuters*, March 11, 2004. Available: http://www.planetark.com/avantgo/dailynewsstory.cfm?newsid=24239. Accessed: March 15, 2004.

Porter, R. *The Greatest Benefit to Mankind*. London: HarperCollins, 1997.

Schwartlander, B., and others. "Resource Needs for HIV/AIDS." *Science*, 2001, *292*(5526), 2434–2436.

World Health Forum. "Highlights of the Early Years Until 1960." *World Health Forum*, 1998, *19*, 24, 21–37.

World Health Organization. *Alma-Ata 1978—Primary Health Care*. Geneva: World Health Organization, 1978.

World Health Organization. *Basic Documents—Forty-fourth edition*. Geneva: World Health Organization, 2003a.

World Health Organization. *World Health Report 2003*. Geneva: World Health Organization, 2003b.

4

Managing Health, Health Care, and Aging

William D. Novelli

The facts and phenomena of aging and health are closely linked. Moreover, they are as "globalized" today as are the realities of trade and economics. The disparities in the quality and delivery of health care between the developed and developing nations in many cases are widening. But given globalization, the rich nations are not immune to health problems found among the poorer nations of the world. Thus, management and leadership for improving global health, especially in an aging world, require an internationalist perspective and, ultimately, worldwide vision and worldwide solutions.

Living in an interconnected world with great disparities in health and health care presents daunting challenges. For example, the persistence and even accelerating spread of human immunodeficiency virus–acquired immunodeficiency syndrome (HIV/AIDS), tuberculosis, and malaria in the poorest nations have both political and social repercussions for wealthier countries. The reemergence of new and sometimes untreatable forms of diseases that the developed world had thought under control—for instance, tuberculosis—underscores that health care problems cannot be settled once and forever but must be solved and then managed with alertness and caution. Modern communications and especially transportation may deliver benefits, such as new therapies that can be announced and delivered with great speed. Yet, emergent diseases, like Ebola virus–caused hemorrhagic fever or severe acute respiratory syndrome (SARS), can hitchhike from continent to continent virtually overnight. Finally, although twenty-five years have passed since the World Health Organization (WHO) presented its Declaration of Alma-Ata, calling for the highest possible standards of health care everywhere in the world, "Health for All" remains a statement of aspiration, not a reality.

The aging of the world's population compounds these problems. Although it is true that many people are living longer and healthier lives, this is chiefly in the developed world. And even in those fortunate countries, the use of medical services among the elderly tends to rise steadily with age. Not too long ago, an optimist could be described as a fifty-year-old person taking out a thirty-year home mortgage. Today, that person might be called a realist. The average life expectancy in the world today is 66 years compared with 46.5 only fifty years ago. In the developed world, longevity is even higher. In the United States, for example, life expectancies are pushing 80 years, and those who live to 65 can expect another eighteen years of life.

Increased longevity is one of the great success stories of the past century, the result of public health measures (including interventions as different as routine vaccinations and improved waste-water treatment), the eradication or at least control of formerly fatal or debilitating childhood diseases, advances in medical knowledge and medical technology, improved diet (although sometimes "improved" to the point of obesity), and higher standards of living, including better education, which tends to run parallel to better health.

These observations should point us toward a new truth about health and age. Old age and ill health have long been considered synonymous. The United Nations Declaration of Human Rights, published in 1948, lumps "old age" in with disability, sickness, and widowhood. This is no longer necessarily the case, especially in the wealthy nations. So we must realize that health is progressive: the health of a child can and often does predict the health of the mature adult. As Alexander Pope (1776, p. 119) put it two centuries ago, "As the twig is bent, so the tree's inclined." We have a longevity bonus, and will continue to live longer, if we cease to think of "child health" as separate from "adult health" and look instead at health just as we look at the entire continuum of life, with each part enabling (or disabling) the next and the next, and so on. Thus, it is important to remember that health can be an absolute itself and not merely the absence of (inevitable) disease or disability. In the same way, we are beginning to understand that age is much more than the residue of youth.

Identifying Challenges in Global Health

What I have just stated grows out of a personal perspective. As the chief executive officer of AARP (formerly the American Association of Retired Persons), the world's largest organization representing older people, I have seen—and will offer more evidence shortly—how health is directly correlated to longevity. Moreover, as former head of the Campaign for Tobacco-Free Kids, I became convinced that what we do when young will, as Pope says, incline us one way or another. Health is important at all ages.

But the longevity bonus also presents us with challenges. More older people in the world will mean more people using more medical services for longer periods. This puts pressures on all nations' economies, most particularly on those with a tradition of legislated health care. Clearly, a public obligation to supply health care directly—or at least health care insurance—will come to compete more and more with other budgetary needs. This can have unpleasant outcomes, including tradeoffs that could make health care less affordable or less accessible for many.

This is not just a future problem: it is already with us. It will simply become more dramatic with time. The World Bank estimates that 16 percent of the world's population, well over a billion men and women, will be aged sixty years or older by 2030. At the same time, birth rates are declining in both developed and developing nations. Thus, by 2050, older people (aged sixty and older) will outnumber children for the first time since the beginning of history. This shift is already noticeable in Europe, which contains twenty-four of the twenty-five "oldest" countries, but not only there; China's population of persons aged sixty and older is expected to climb from 10 percent today to 22 percent by 2030. Besides the budgetary problems mentioned earlier, this presents the possibility of pitting generation against generation for what they want from national resources. Young people may see subsidized higher education as a greater benefit than subsidized health care, whereas older people might see it the other way around.

Thus, addressing the dramatically rising cost of delivering health care and maintaining health is a key challenge for leaders. According to AARP's research, several factors affect health as we age. Clearly, health in earlier life, as previously noted, is crucial. Even so, some factors continue to drive up costs, some as a consequence of individual choice but others beyond any individual control. For example, some things that drive health care costs upward are persistent low levels of physical activity among older people; exercise as simple as walking on a regular basis can improve cardiovascular health; weight training, even done in a swimming pool, can strengthen bones and improve disorders of the joints. Another cost-driving factor is the development of new and generally expensive medicines and medical technologies. These in turn lead to medical inflation, which routinely outpaces general consumer price increases, sometimes by two to one or more.

And the amounts at issue are considerable. The Organization for Economic Cooperation and Development (OECD) estimates that health spending averages 9 percent of the gross domestic product (GDP) in the OECD area—twice what it was in 1970. It further predicts that spending on health in relation to GDP will rise by 50 to 60 percent by the middle of the century. The United States has already arrived at that level, spending 15.3 percent of GDP on health today, with expectations that it will grow at about 7 percent annually (whereas general inflation is under 3 percent), reaching $2.8 trillion by 2011. But the overall pinch on governments will be somewhat comparable: *public* spending on health in the United States, along with Mexico and Korea, represents less than half of *total* health expenses, but in the OECD countries the average is more than 70 percent.

This is really a matter of cost shifting. According to the European Commission and OECD, *public* spending on health benefits for the elderly in a typical developed country will grow from 11 percent to 18 percent of GDP over the next fifty years. Furthermore, because some three-quarters of all health spending in OECD countries is dependent on public financing, the decrease of the working-age population and the resultant weakening of the tax base will provide additional strain on governments as they continue to provide effective and affordable health care to their citizens. One reason for this quandary is that the Western European democracies have been reluctant or at least slow to require more contribution toward costs from individuals, although this may be changing. In the United States, on the other hand, out-of-pocket spending on prescription drugs and long-term care represents a great financial issue for older Americans. Out-of-pocket health costs average 19 percent of income for persons aged sixty-five and older in the United States.

This may reflect both cultural and political differences between Europe and America. In Europe, I often hear from experts who consider the American health care system out of balance for leaving millions of uninsured while spending more than any other country on health care. Out-of-pocket expenses in other G8 countries are lower because these nations often use a universal, predominantly publicly funded health care model that often sets specific limits on health spending. For patients, however, this can mean long waits for services or policies that prevent anyone over a certain age from receiving expensive treatments, such as coronary bypass surgery or a hip replacement. On the other hand, in the United States, elderly patients have elective surgeries that would be denied to them in other countries. In fact, wealthy elderly Europeans come to the United States for treatments that are simply not available to them because of the severity of their disorders or their age.

Although the problems of medical costs, quality, and access vary from country to country, it is clear that they grow out of personal behavior or expectation and out of government policy. Consequently, leaders facing the pressures of health care quality and delivery in an aging world need to look for means to alter individual expectations and behaviors and also systems and public policies. This is beginning to happen, albeit slowly and irregularly. For example, in Germany patients used to show their insurance card and never expected to see a bill. Now the government has altered the structure of the "sickness fund" so that patients will have a "co-pay" for prescription drugs, dental treatments, and hospitalizations. In Japan, the government has proposed cutbacks for in-home nursing care services for the elderly, which could affect 1.7 million older Japanese. Whether this is the wisest way to save money—care at home can often be cheaper than care in hospitals or formal health care settings—remains to be seen. To assist vulnerable U.S. citizens with out-of-pocket drug costs, the U.S. government passed a $400 billion bill to include prescription drug coverage through Medicare. AARP supported this bill because it will help millions of older people pay the high cost of their medications. But we also recognized that it is only a foundation on which to build and improve. So we are pursuing a wide range of federal, state, and consumer initiatives to make prescription drugs more affordable. These include educating consumers on steps they can take to make their health care dollars go further.

Policymakers and other leaders need to find innovative solutions to the problem of high health care costs that go beyond limiting access and shifting costs among the government, individuals, and business. For example, we need to examine how pharmaceutical corporations develop their pricing structures while seeing what can be done to enable these companies to bring their therapies to market at lower prices without compromising safety and efficacy. This would certainly require leadership by both the private and the public sectors.

One of the key challenges we face is in long-term care and disease management. Much of our health care system is focused on care for acute conditions, but chronic conditions are growing more common as people age, and treating them is eating up a larger and larger portion of our health budget.

Such conditions, including heart disease, diabetes, and asthma, are now the leading causes of illness, disability, and death. But today's health system remains overly devoted to dealing with acute, episodic conditions. Our health care system is seriously lacking in clinical programs with the multidisciplinary infrastructure required to provide the full complement of services needed by people with common chronic conditions.

The fact that more than 40 percent of people with chronic conditions have more than one such condition argues strongly for more sophisticated mechanisms to coordinate care. Yet, health care organizations, hospitals, and physician groups typically operate as separate "silos," acting without the benefit of complete information about a patient's condition, medical history, services provided in other settings, or medications provided by other clinicians.

The Centers for Disease Control and Prevention (CDC) report that chronic diseases, such as heart disease, cancer, and diabetes, are the leading causes of death and disability in the United States. They account for seven of every ten deaths and affect the quality of life of ninety million Americans. However, although chronic diseases are among the most common and costly health problems, they are also among the most preventable.

The American Diabetes Association, for example, estimates the costs of diabetes care at $132 billion annually, and much of that money comes from Medicare and Medicaid. So it is important that we not only help people by making their drugs more affordable but also help them to better manage chronic diseases such as diabetes.

Although we need to do much more to prevent the onset of chronic diseases, we must also find better ways to treat and manage them. In Medicare, for example, costly beneficiaries are likely to have multiple chronic conditions. One analysis found that beneficiaries with three or more conditions (46 percent of beneficiaries) account for almost 90 percent of total spending whereas those with no chronic conditions account for less than 1 percent (Anderson, 2004). Furthermore, about half the cost in any one year for Medicare is due to 5 percent of the beneficiaries—those with multiple chronic conditions. Today we are not doing enough to manage that care and contain those costs.

We should focus on better management of such conditions, on controlling them with exercise, diet, and medication rather than intervening with hospitalizations and surgeries. The importance of this change of approach is becoming more pressing all the time because more than half of America's baby boomers will live to see their eighty-fifth birthdays—and no doubt multiple chronic conditions. The same will be happening virtually everywhere in the world. Fortunately, the new Medicare law contains important provisions for chronic disease management.

Opportunities for Leadership

Addressing costs and access is just the beginning. Identifying and exploiting ideas and opportunities to keep improving both health and health care are just as important. Emphasis should be on improving health and health care, not just health care by itself. There are many ways people can live healthier lives without resorting to the particular health care system of which they are a part. Certainly emphasizing preventive health is critical, and this does call into play the health care system, usually in the form of screenings (especially for breast, prostate, and colorectal cancer), regular checkups, flu shots, and so forth. Preventive health has the advantage of avoiding future bottlenecks and future higher costs for more elaborate interventions.

But it is also important to look at health as an individual matter. A focus on healthy living from childhood, as previously noted, creates healthier lives later on, which in turn means older people may continue to contribute to society and reduce the strain on health care systems and on their own budgets. What starts early pays off later. Duane Alexander (2001) of the U.S. National Institute for Child Health and Human Development, part of the National Institutes of Health, commented, "Osteoporosis is a pediatric disease with geriatric consequences." This is worth expanding on: Most teenaged girls and about half of teenaged boys do not get enough calcium at a time when they are acquiring 90 percent of the bone mass they will ever have. The result of weaker bones is more fractures, more joint problems, and more disability for individuals and more costs for health care. Drinking milk—and it can be nonfat— at age fourteen can pay off well at age seventy-four. The same is true of other behavioral aspects of health, including never smoking and controlling weight. These and other health-promoting and disease-preventing efforts have a tremendous effect on one's quality of life throughout the life span.

There are other examples. Research shows that adult afflictions like heart disease and high blood pressure frequently have origins in early childhood behaviors. Lack of fitness, apart from contributing to being overweight, brings on its own problems, including a slowed metabolism, depression, brittleness of bones, and poor circulation. A study reported in the *New England Journal of Medicine* found that poor physical fitness is a better predictor of death than any other risk factor, including smoking, high blood pressure, and heart disease (Myers and others, 2002).

We have all seen headlines calling obesity the "new epidemic of our century." In 1991, 22 percent of Americans were obese. The number has increased to over 30 percent, and the projection for

2025 is 42 percent (National Center for Health Statistics, 2003). Although the United States has one of the highest rates of obesity in the world, obesity is increasing in other countries as well. Currently, one child in ten worldwide is overweight. Studies show that eating habits and obesity can affect the risk for premature cancer, diabetes, liver and heart diseases, and many other problems. Therefore, it is important to recognize that eating behavior and food preferences, key determinants of long-term health, are primarily established in childhood. According to the Pediatric Clinics of America, 80 percent of children who are overweight grow into obese adults (Lakdawalla, Bhattacharya, and Goldman, 2004). We have an opportunity to reverse this trend by encouraging healthy living, beginning at an early age.

It is equally important to promote the concept of "healthy aging," including stressing good diet and exercise later in life. Ohio State University researchers found that older people who exercise regularly are more likely to maintain brain function used for everyday tasks, like following a recipe or remembering the right doses of medications they take every day. These are enormous and positive implications of good health that can bring important benefits for the population as it ages (Emery and others, 2003).

Although bad habits are not broken overnight, we have evidence that they can be successfully influenced over time. In 1964, the U.S. Surgeon General warned about the dangers of smoking cigarettes, spurring a campaign of warning messages everywhere (National Centers for Disease Control and Prevention, 1964). Although few people quit immediately, more and more have over time or never started smoking at all. Adult smoking is down by over 50 percent, leading to a decline in the incidence of lung cancer and emphysema.

Improvements in diet, smoking cessation, seat-belt use, and greater fitness prove that it is possible for attitudes and behaviors to change, although the obesity epidemic will be a great challenge. But, clearly, change is possible. So we must promote a new point of view, a new mind-set of attitudes toward aging. First, aging is not and should not be synonymous with disability. Second, health is not something that is applied—although health care is—but is maintained and promoted throughout one's life. And third, a productive, positive lifestyle is possible for most people at virtually any age.

We must look more at the continuum of life, not at magic numbers like forty for middle age, sixty-five for retirement, and so on, because the numbers themselves have little meaning. More healthy older people, regardless of their age, will provide more mentors, caregivers, and volunteers in the societies of tomorrow. Healthy aging also unleashes the creative powers of people who, despite their age, have lost none of their intelligence and have added years of experience, even hard knocks, along the way to help them solve problems. Healthy aging can also unlock the commercial and consumer powers held by older people, especially if they keep working and earning.

We can look forward to societies where second and third careers are routine and where companies can find experienced workers without having to look abroad. These are goals we can achieve, although we have a long way to go. In Japan, 45 percent of men and 20 percent of woman older than sixty still work. In America, it is only 23 percent of men and 13 percent of women, and in France, just 6 percent of men and 4 percent of women still are in the workforce. Imagine if these numbers were to grow in proportion to greater health and longevity; imagine how this would reduce the pressure of health care costs, expand the tax base (including payments to Social Security and Medicare from those who are already its beneficiaries), and give older people the income and sense of accomplishment that many will want.

The nations of the world can learn from one another about sustaining and applying both healthy behavior and health care across the life span. Shifting focus to prevention from treatment and from acute interventions to long-term treatments can moderate costs (whether the public sector or the individual pays does not matter in this case: money saved is money saved) and provide the more appropriate kind of care. For example, the transformation of the U.S. Veterans Health Administration's approach from hospital to ambulatory care in the 1990s helped reduce expenditures per patient about 25 percent (Perlin, Kolodner, and Roswell, 2004).

The CamCare project in the Netherlands, developed with subsidies from the Ministry of Health, provides medical advice and information to homebound patients with audio and video links (*Health Beat*, 2004). Response is quick and costs are negligible because there is no visit to a physician's office or a house call for a medical worker to make. There are other ways to practice "e-medicine," especially for routine questions between physician and patient. We will learn to apply technology to connect patients, physicians, general health information, pharmacists, and so forth—at a fraction of current costs.

Need for Leadership and Global Collaboration

The desire for good health and access to health care knows no borders. One cannot speak of global health and ignore the tragedy of disease and epidemics in the poor world. A WHO study (2001) confirmed that extreme poverty in the world stems in great part from the lack of adequate health services. Sick people cannot contribute economically or socially. These health care conditions and the challenges of bankrupt governments, collapsed economies, and failed states demand a global commitment, led by the developed world, to provide more resources and attention to the health care plight of poor countries.

Beyond altruism, we should recognize that investment in health care in the poor countries will offer good returns in the form of peace and stability around the world. First of all, improving health—and especially the delivery of health care to the young— in the developing world will slow population growth. According to Columbia University's Jeffrey D. Sachs (2002), poor people have smaller families when they know their children will not die young or at birth.

Global health is not only a matter of the rich nations helping the poor. With the growing maturity of the European Union (EU) and with more and more migration and guest workers around the world, international cooperation and consultation have already become facts of life. The recent expansion of the EU will have major implications for the way health care is provided. Citizens of EU member states were presented with an EU health card at the beginning of 2004, allowing them easier access to health care services across the EU. However, there are already discrepancies among various national health systems, and therefore, the need to standardize services across all member states is obvious. International consultation and cooperation will be necessary to assure that the provision of health care across all of the EU adheres to the same high standards.

The EU, like WHO and the OECD, are useful international forums for defining the problems and challenges of health and aging on a global level and provide useful ideas or modalities to individual nations. We can use transnational organizations, like WHO, and even private organizations like the Red Cross, CARE, and Doctors Without Borders, to exchange ideas and information from one country to another. We should encourage and support such organizations. This returns us to an earlier theme: that we have much to learn from each other.

For example, American policymakers have been observing the consumer-directed home care programs developed in Europe that rely on consumers, rather than public agencies, to hire, train, and supervise home care workers. The Netherlands, Germany, and the United Kingdom have already had good results by changing the nature of noninstitutional services so that people with disabilities have more control over the services they require.

This is all good news, but many goals remain far off as we deal with the facts of life and especially of politics. It would be wonderful if there were, in America and elsewhere in the world, bipartisan or rather nonpartisan agreement about the role of government in health care, about what costs are sustainable by government and by individuals, and about the standards of high-quality health care. This will require aggressive leadership and active collaboration from all corners of society. We will need the participation of the legislative and executive branches of government, of government-supported health research organizations, of pharmaceutical and biotechnology firms and other corporations, and of nongovernmental organizations, foundations, private philanthropy, advocacy groups, and citizen activists.

The goals of such collaborative effort will differ from country to country. But such a broad spectrum of cooperation could defuse some of the political and commercial bickering over resource allocation and advance ideas that indirectly reduce health care costs (health promotion and disease prevention). Selling reductions in benefits or higher out-of-pocket costs would be more difficult. Besides national debates, international discussions and collaboration could reduce some of the political heat and fallout from suggestions that may not have large natural constituencies in any one country.

I began by saying that the facts and phenomena of health and aging are closely linked and global. Why, then, should our responses to the challenges they present us not also be global? We have much to learn from one another as societies and economies become more closely linked.

Improving global health is not simply a question of know-how or technology. We have much of the knowledge and the tools. It is a question of political will, establishing priorities and allocating resources—that is, of deciding to apply our know-how and technology. It is also a question of taking a collaborative view of the world and our problems and recognizing that we are all in this together. In other words, improving global health truly will require cooperation and far-sighted leadership.

References

Alexander, D. "'Calcium Crisis' Affects American Youth." Press Release. Rockville, Md.: National Institute of Child Health and Human Development, Dec. 10, 2001. Available: www.nichd.nih.gov/new/releases/calcium_crisis.cfm.

Anderson, G. "Partnership for Solutions: Better Lives for People with Chronic Conditions." *Report to the Congress: Medicare Payment Policy*. Washington, D.C.: MEDPAC. Available: www.medpac.gov. Accessed: March 2004.

Emery, C. F., and others. "Cognitive and Psychological Outcomes of Exercise in a 1-Year Follow-up Study of Patients with Chronic Obstructive Pulmonary Disease," *Health Psychology*, Nov. 2003, *22*(6), 598–604.

Health Beat. "Dutch Home Care Project Remotely Connects Patients to Providers," *Health Beat*, May 13, 2004. Available: www.ihealthbeat.org/index.cfm?Action=dspItem&itemID=102725.

Lakdawalla, D. N., Bhattacharya, J., and Goldman, D. P. "Are the Young Becoming More Disabled? Rates of Disability Appear to Be on the Rise Among People Ages Eighteen to Fifty-Nine, Fueled by a Growing Obesity Epidemic," *Health Affairs*, Jan./Feb. 2004, *23*(1), 168–176.

Myers, J., and others. "Exercise Capacity and Mortality Among Men Referred for Exercise Testing." *New England Journal of Medicine*, March 14, 2002, *346*, 793–801.

National Centers for Disease Control and Prevention. *1964 Surgeon General Report: Reducing the Health Consequences of Smoking*. Washington, D.C.: U.S. Government Printing Office, 1964. Available: www.cdc.gov/tobacco/sgr/sgr_1964/sgr64.htm.

National Center for Health Statistics. *Health, United States, 2003*. Washington, D.C.: U.S. Government Printing Office, Oct. 2003.

Perlin, J. B., Kolodner, R. M., and Roswell, R. H. "The Veterans Health Administration: Quality, Value, Accountability, and Information as Transforming Strategies for Patient-Centered Care," *The American Journal of Managed Care*, Nov. 2004, pp. 828–836.

Pope, A. "Epistle I: To Sir Richard Temple, Lord Cobham," *Moral Essays*. London: William Banes, 1776.

Sachs, J. D. *Scaling Up the Responses to Infectious Diseases: A Way out of Poverty*. Geneva: World Health Organization, 2002. Available: www.who/int/infectious-disease-report/2002/pdfversion/Ch2HealthServices.pdf.

World Health Organization, Commission on Macroeconomics and Health. *Macroeconomics and Health: Investing in Health for Economic Development*. Geneva: World Health Organization, Dec. 2001.

Part II

Developing Strategies,
New Pathways, and Solutions

5

Leadership, Equity, and Global Health

Harlan Cleveland

Half a century ago, in company with journalist-historian Theodore H. White, I spent an evening with Victor Weisskopf, one of the physicists who worked on the world's first nuclear weapons. What I remember most vividly is not what he said about physics or the Bomb.

As we wound up our interview, I asked him whether, if he were to start all over again, he would be a physicist. "No, I'd want to be a biologist," he replied without hesitation. After a pause, his face broke into a smile of pure delight. "What a wonderful field! They don't know anything yet. They don't know what life is. They don't know what goes on inside a cell." The life scientists still do not claim to know just what life is or why; they cannot even agree when it starts. But they *are* learning what goes on inside a cell and even how to modify its function, change its behavior.

Nature and nurture, which used to be separately taught and studied, have come together in molecular biology. Genetic engineers are learning how to move genes in and out of species. Computer experts are stretching the limits of speed and memory to map

Portions of this chapter were derived from Koop, Pearson, and Schwarz (2002); McHale and McHale (1978); and Cleveland (1985, 1997). See Cleveland (2002) for further discussion of leadership trends.

the whole of the human genome. Scientists have married genetics and chemistry to begin to decipher our most powerful information system, the one we are born with. As Weisskopf foresaw, the biologists and their friends are having a ball.

And in the new branch of engineering called biotechnology, they are enabling us—human beings, *homo* we hope *sapiens*—to mastermind our own evolution.

It is an exhilarating assignment—and a scary one. The people who started the Scientific Revolution—Copernicus, Galileo, Newton, and the rest—surely did not foresee that in a few centuries, people might generate the knowledge and acquire the capacity to do more to their natural environment than Nature does to, and for, people. Yet, this is where we are headed today. An ironic anonymous couplet says it all:

> Strange that man should make up lists of living things
> in danger.
> Why he fails to list himself is really even stranger.

So let us explore the strange, and changing, environment for global health.

Management of Ourselves

In the slices of health literature a generalist can absorb, I am impressed by how much of "world health" breaches the boundaries of "health systems." One of the *Critical Issues* papers, by Kumi Naidoo, says that "only about 10 percent of potential [health] improvements in developed countries will come from advances in health technology and management. Almost half will come from preventive personal health practices. And half will come from improvements in the environment we provide for human life" (2002, p. 408).

The logic is clear enough. Our biggest problem is not so much the management of world health, important and difficult as that already is. The transcendent puzzle is the management of ourselves, of the human actions and inactions that are by far the largest component of the health of humans.

As we awaken to this new awareness, we can see ahead a new class of problems, requiring unprecedented kinds of solutions:

They Are Global

They require people everywhere to widen to world scale what they worry about and try to do something about. Dean Abrahamson, a hard-science colleague at the University of Minnesota, had a graphic way of saying this: "When my grandfather was born, environmental concerns were almost all based on housekeeping and trash in the backyard. By the time I was born, there were demonstrable regional impacts. The birth of my children coincided with entire river systems and airsheds being affected. Now major global systems, upon which society depends for its welfare, are being destroyed" (personal communication).

They Are Behavioral

Global health is now mostly the sum of what billions of individuals—and hundreds of millions of couples—are doing or failing to do. Its pace and direction will mostly be changed by what all those individuals and couples do, and stop doing, next. Réné Dubos had it right many years ago: "Think globally, act locally."

The threats to health systems are daunting enough, even if they are only one-tenth of our health futures. Two of them seem especially worth highlighting before we move on.

One is the speed with which the elderly nearly everywhere are getting older. Folks older than eighty-five are clearly winning the population growth rate derby. Now that I have myself passed that magic number, I cannot manage to feel as gloomy about it as some young demographers do.

Indeed, I am now inclined to question the extreme preoccupation of medical and social policy with the "frail elderly." At least in the United States, public policy has focused mostly on those (probably less than 20 percent of those in "the third stage of life") who are unable to cope without continuous support systems—hospitals, nursing homes, assisted living, special transportation, home-delivered meals, live-in nurses—and a growing need for public subsidies.

I am far from suggesting neglect of this compassionate end of the scale. Indeed, I am grateful for the U.S. taxpayer's willingness to pay sizable chunks of my own impressive medical bills. But I think that each of our national societies needs to devote much more time, attention, and imagination to what Robert Butler calls the productive aging of the other 80 percent or more, the elderly and coping. Twenty years ago, well before my own chronology induced a serious interest in policies about aging, I wrote this comment on the social value of longevity in an information society:

> Now, who is likely to be best qualified for the kind of work that is heavy with personal relations, integrative thinking, and reflective action? Who are the most natural members of the get-it-all-together profession? Who are the people among us with the most experience in solving unprecedented problems, the people most likely to have seen more of the world, mastered or at least dabbled in more specialties, learned to distinguish the candor from the cant in corporate and bureaucratic life and in public affairs, the people with the most time for reflection and the most to reflect about? The answer leaps to

the eye: They are, on the average, those who have lived longer (Cleveland, 1985, p. 217).

The other current health threat that leaps to the eye is what Professor Ramalingaswami (2002) called "a double burden . . . high rates of infectious diseases with rising rates of chronic noncommunicable diseases" (p. 62). We do not get to choose between these two burdens. As soon as she became director general of the World Health Organization (WHO), Gro Harlem Brundtland of Norway laid down as a basic principle that these are not competing tasks. They are complementary. We need to fight both. The burden of disease is the burden of unfulfilled human development. They are not just complementary; they may even be mutually reinforcing. Future studies may well demonstrate infectious disease connections to everything from arthritis to mental illness.

Coping with infectious disease brings us to the double trouble with immunization. We are reminded again and again about the propensity of microorganisms to "fulfill their Darwinian destiny" by designing their ways around the drugs we throw at them—and which we use or misuse in quantities that help build resistance to them. As if that were not enough, William H. Foege (2002, p. 116) has written that "the HIV [human immunodeficiency virus] literally disarmed us by taking a new evolutionary step, attacking the very system designed to provide us protection."

Speaking as an amateur, I find it hard to receive professional news like this with equanimity. But I want now to sketch the future of world health as part of a broader canvas, which may help us get our rethinking started well short of the "slough of despond."

On that broader canvas, let us consider four pieces of a common puzzle: the interlocked complexity of "basic human needs," the impact (on health and everything else) of the information revolution, its implications (in health and everything else) for fairness and equity, and the new requirements (in health and everything else) for leadership.

Basic Human Needs

The health of humans is mostly not the product of medical procedures and professional caregiving to cure or prevent disease in individuals—important, indeed essential, as these are. It is the product of their environment, which may mean their physical surround (living conditions, poisonous water, polluted air, and so on) or their social conditions (poverty, malnutrition, sour relationships)—and their personal behavior (smoking, fast driving, unsafe sex, or whatever).

In this context, nutrition can be seen as an environmental factor, as can housing, clothing, and population growth. And so can educational attainment, especially of women whose understanding of reproduction and the care and cure of children is usually the make-or-break factor in infant mortality and the healthy development of children.

When in 1948 the United Nations tried to express global entitlements in a Universal Declaration of Human Rights (Eleanor Roosevelt was a prime mover in its negotiation), health naturally had to be edited into a complicated mix:

> **Article 25**
> 1. Everyone has the right to a standard of living adequate for the health and well-being of himself and his family, including food, clothing, housing, and medical care and necessary social services, and the right to security in the event of unemployment, sickness, disability, widowhood, old age, or other lack of livelihood in circumstances beyond his control (United Nations, 1950).

When in the 1970s I worked with John and Magda McHale to find a way to describe basic human needs worldwide, we found no ready-made analytical framework for defining, targeting, and measuring each category of need. "Health" had to be stirred together with poverty, nutrition, education, family planning, employment, compensation for accidents, retirement schemes, "and such collective entitlements as mass transit, air and water quality standards, parks and recreation areas, and more or less limited rights to travel, to be informed, to assemble, to speak and to participate in community decisions" (Cleveland, 1978, p. 11).

The assessment of needs not only varied by climate, diet, income, and education, but most of the measuring sticks commonly used in the field of health focused not on people's health but on the capacity of societies to handle illness—that is, the health of the health delivery system. In similar manner, educational achievement is still often expressed as the number of years a person has spent in a formal course of study, rather than what the student may have learned in school or from life experience.

Longevity, the measuring stick often used as a rough measure of a population's health, does by its nature take into account many factors beyond the delivery of health services. But by sweeping into a statistical blender such numbers as people killed in wars or on highways, the length of life is hardly a sensitive instrument for measuring a population's health and well-being.

The 1978 McHale and McHale report, prepared for the U.N. Environmental Program, was an exhaustive analysis, "casting physical needs up against availabilities of resources . . . in a 'balance of things' rather than a fiscal budget or a balance of payments,"—with an upbeat conclusion: "Absolute poverty is due not to shortfalls of material or technological resources but to shortcomings of social imagination and political management. Minimum human needs can in fact be met worldwide, by a generation of relevant and cooperative effort" (Cleveland, 1978, pp. 16, 19).

This judgment is even more valid in the first decade of the twenty-first century than it was nearly thirty years ago. As applied to health, the reason is precisely that, as the *Basic Human Needs* report put it, "health care is essentially social."

Symbols, Not Things

The recent celebrations of the third millennium brought a flood of commentary about the horrors and delights awaiting us just ahead. In trying to think about the next few decades, I was struck by the extent to which all the observable trends were rooted in the historically sudden spread of knowledge, which in turn is the consequence of upheavals and opportunities created by the marriage of computers and telecommunications during the last quarter of the twentieth century.

Peering now into the twenty-first century, we cannot know just what will happen or when. But we already know something more important: why it will happen.

Information—symbols, not things—will clearly be playing the lead role in world history that physical labor, stone, bronze, land, minerals, and energy once played. We will have to burn into our consciousness how different information is from all its predecessors as civilization's dominant resource.

Information *expands as it is used*—no limits to growth here. It is readily *transportable*, at close to the speed of light—and much faster than that. Information *leaks* so easily that it is much harder to hide and to hoard than tangible resources were. The spread of knowledge *empowers the many* by eroding the influence that once empowered the few who were "in the know." Information *cannot be owned*; only its delivery service can. And *giving or selling information* does not give rise to "exchange" transactions; they are acts of sharing.

These six simple, pregnant propositions, as they sink in and around the world and down the generations, should help us sort out some of the big conundrums that puzzle us as we turn the corner to a new millennium.

For example: One offspring of that great social event of the 1980s—the marriage of computers and telecommunications—is the changing relevance of distance.

Down through history, "community" has mostly meant the ties among people who lived or worked near each other. Even where a community's roots were rooted in a common religion or ethnic identity, people identified most closely with the like-minded who were geographically close at hand. But now and in the future, the comparative ease of travel and communication makes it much easier for community to mean people with similar interests and motivations working together in "virtual teams" wherever they are living, working, or even traveling.

It is certainly premature, but it is no longer laughable, to speak of "the end of geography." With electronics, satellites, and fast computers at our command, we have all watched the dwindling relevance of distance in our intellectual pursuits. But we also noticed that delivering facts and ideas, which can be done efficiently from a distance, is only half of teaching-learning dynamics. The other half is "getting to know you, getting to know all about you"—the magic, human, and social part of education.

Computer-assisted communication is not a substitute for face-to-face contact, but the converse is equally true. Once I get to know you pretty well, up close and personal, I really do not need to see your face every time we talk on the phone or exchange messages by e-mail. What is clear is that combining up-close and distance learning enhances the educational experience beyond what is possible with either mode alone.

It will be interesting to see whether, in thinking about the dwindling of distance, the professions of medicine and public health reach for a comparable synthesis. Of course, some of the great successes in public health—the eradication of smallpox is an obvious example—have been enabled by the wide spread of knowledge, plus intensive international cooperation. And the codification and communication of best practices in everything from diagnostics to surgery is already proving to be a bonanza in the treatment of disease in the remotest places.

But does that mean, as a "Human Genome Survey" four years ago in *The Economist* came close to suggesting under the provocative subhead "Move Over Hippocrates," that the physician's role will be superseded by automated expert systems, "by chips of one sort or another"? ("Human Genome Survey," 2000).

I hope and believe it is much more likely that, in health as in other professions, automated skills and distance delivery will still require sensitive professionals to interpret, for real-life patients and the families they have come to know personally, the novel insights that new information technologies will make both possible and globally accessible.

Global Fairness Revolution

Yet another consequence of the pervasive information revolution is a sudden change in the global prospects for fairness. I was impressed four years ago by how often in the *Critical Issues* volume authors would complain about inequity in global health, then stop short of prescribing remedies for it.

"The poor and marginalized are the major health challenge the world faces," wrote Nils Daulaire. "The world of the twenty-first century could become a world more deeply split into disparate health groups, with the medical 'haves' achieving life expectancies approaching a century while the medical 'have-nots' struggle to reach and maintain half that" (2002, p. 426). The intervening years have only confirmed that astute forecast. The most memorable, and most succinct, summation of health in the twentieth century was that of Foege: "spectacular achievements, spectacular inequities."

Poor health is above all a function of poverty; that is clear enough from the record of civilizations so far. A doleful legacy of the twentieth century is the still-growing gap between rich and poor, among countries and inside countries. As information—abundant, shareable, and instantly accessible—now becomes the world's dominant resource, what will that do to the prospects for fairness?

Surely it means that people who get educated to handle information, who hone their analytical and intuitive powers, who learn how to achieve access to information, and even more important, how to select what they need for the information overload will likely be better off and more fairly treated than those who do not.

In the industrial era, poverty was explained and justified by shortages of things; there just were not enough minerals, food, fiber, and manufactures to go around. Looked at this way, the resource shortages were merely aggravated by the propensity of the poor to have babies.

In the era just ahead of us, physical resources are elbowed from center stage by information, the resource that is hardest for the rich and powerful to hide or hoard. Each of the babies, poor or not, is born with a brain. The collective capacity of all the brains in each society to convert information into knowledge and wisdom is the measure of that society's potential. Consider this measuring rod as you think about China's role—and India's, too—in the twenty-first century.

But there is a catch: Whether the "informatization" of the globe will actually mean a fairer shake for those who in earlier times have been the victims of discrimination depends mostly on what *they* do from now on.

Most of the fairness achieved in world history has not been the consequence of charity, good-heartedness, or noblesse oblige on the part of those who already possessed riches and power. Always in history, it seems, fairness has been granted, legislated, or seized when there was no alternative. Usually the reason there was no alternative was that the "downs" were determined, or at least feared by the "ups" to be determined, to cast off their shackles and take the law into their own hands.

As information leaks around the world, a large number of people are now learning, often instantly, about what goes on elsewhere: good things happening in places near and far that could happen to them if their leaders were wiser and more flexible and bad things happening to other people that could fall out on them if they do not watch out.

During the revolutions of 1989–1991 that pulled the fraying rugs from under the Communist regimes of Eastern Europe, then swept into history the Soviet Union itself, the impatient crowds in the big public squares were moved not by distant visions of utopia but by readily accessible information about neighbors in Western Europe who were obviously getting more goods and services, more fairness in their distribution, and firmer guarantees of human rights than their own bosses and planners seemed able to deliver.

The good news was that information leaked—and that sharing has long been the natural mode of scientific and cultural communication. The changing information environment was bound to undermine the knowledge monopolies that totalitarian governments had converted into monopolies of power.

The learners in every society are starting to fashion their own road signs, some resulting from experiments derived from what the West has shown is possible, some adapted and updated from older systems of wisdom, and some the result of new intellectual or spiritual inspiration.

The more affluent countries—and the more affluent people in every country—thus face a global fairness revolution, multiplying the demands on a world economic system that still shares its benefits with only a minority of humankind.

Both among and within the "nation-states" of the twenty-first century, the old French warning retains its relevance: *Entre le fort et le faible, c'est la liberté qui opprime et la loi qui affranchit* ("In relations between the strong and the weak, it is freedom that oppresses and law that liberates"). But if law is too rigid and universal, as Aristotle had already figured out two-and-a-half millennia ago, the urge for equity or fairness will arise to correct the law. Part of the stew of resentments seems always to be the complaint every child learns to make from infancy: "It isn't fair."

The key that unlocks "growth with fairness," in the United States and elsewhere in the global information society, is widespread access to relevant education.

More than any one factor, it was that forward-looking early-nineteenth-century decision to mandate free public education for every young U.S. resident that enabled the American people to pull themselves out of "underdevelopment." Another wise educational policy, the Morrill Act of 1862, used federal land grants to set up university-based agricultural research stations and build a county-by-county extension service to deliver the resulting science directly to farmers. That made possible those "amber waves of grain," celebrated in our loveliest national song, that are still today a centerpiece of the world food market.

Around the horizon of the developing world—in Asia, Africa, and Latin America—the close connection between education and equitable development is now crystal clear: *The poor can get rich by brain work.*

The Japanese amply illustrated this theorem of wealth creation from the earliest dawn of the information era. Two of the most dramatic demonstrations in my lifetime have been India's Green Revolution in the 1970s, a public-sector initiative, and the private-sector software surge in the 1990s that has made India a global player in the world's most phenomenal new industry.

Also in my own lifetime, the hustling people of South Korea, empowered and emboldened by a national policy of universal education dating only from the 1950s, have now become the newest members of the Organization for Economic Cooperation and Development (OECD), the "rich countries" club. During the same half-century, Taiwan, Singapore, and Israel have in their differing ways demonstrated the close connections between brainpower and prosperity. Not only have their economies grown faster than those in most other developing countries, but also the benefits of that growth have been spread more fairly among their own people than in developing countries that are "favored" (as they are not) by endowments of oil, hard minerals, good soil, or moderate climate.

The growing importance of brain work has to be good news for every country less endowed with geological riches and arable farmland than were the early arrivers of the industrial age. Around the developing world, the striking paradox is that the most successful countries are precisely those not blessed with wealth-creating natural resources.

By contrast, in the countries whose people have been kept in ignorance (by colonial policies or their own leaders' mismanagement, or first one and then the other), it hardly seems to matter what riches lie in the space they occupy. Most of their citizens become peasants of the information society, along with the dropouts in the postindustrial world. The physical riches get siphoned off to benefit educated folk huddling in the affluent sections of their central cities and to enrich the information-wise foreigners who "come to do good, and do well."

Twilight of Hierarchy

To chart the potentials of the global information revolution is not to fulfill them. The predictable trends in information technology will make it possible to organize as a commons most of the world's most useful health information, serving it up to those on every continent who take the trouble and make the effort to convert it into usable knowledge and practical wisdom. But how will this get done? And who will lead in the doing of it?

To clarify my answer to these questions, I have to expose readers to my way of thinking about the shifting seismology of organization and leadership. The direction of change is now more than obvious: everywhere, a shift from top-down "vertical" relationships toward "horizontal," consensual, and collaborative modes of bringing people together.

This major historical fault line is also clearly a consequence of the spread of information—symbols, not things—as the newly dominant resource. The more people are in the know, empowered by ready access to the enormous pool of knowledge available through the Internet, worldwide journals, and global radio and television, the more likely they are to think they have something relevant to say— and to insist on being heard.

It was in the nature of *things* that the few had access to key resources and the many did not; there never seemed to be enough to go around. The inherent characteristics of physical resources (the natural ones and those created by human ingenuity) made possible, perhaps even necessary, the development of hierarchies: hierarchies of *power based on control* (of new weapons, of transport vehicles, of trade routes, of markets, and even of knowledge back when knowing could be kept private), hierarchies of *influence based on secrecy*, hierarchies of *class based on ownership*, hierarchies of *privilege based on early access* to particular pieces of land or especially valuable resources, and hierarchies of *politics based on geography*.

Each of these five bases for hierarchy and discrimination was crumbling in the waning years of the twentieth century. The old means of control are of dwindling efficacy. Secrets are harder and harder to keep (as the Central Intelligence Agency and the White House relearn every few weeks). And ownership, early arrival, and geography are of declining importance in accessing, remembering, analyzing, and using the knowledge and wisdom that are the valuable legal tender of our time.

The twilight of hierarchy opens up a fast-growing need for people who can and will take the lead—and requires different attitudes and strategies for those who opt to point the way. In modern societies, many organizations still look from a distance like pyramids, but both their internal processes and their external relations feature much less order-giving and much more consultation and consensus.

(Consensus is *not* the same as "unanimous consent." When I was practicing diplomacy at the United Nations and in NATO, I found helpful this definition of the word *consensus*: the acquiescence of those who care [about each particular decision], supported by the apathy of those who do not.)

Nobody in Charge

This seismic shift that is making the administrative pyramid obsolete has now been going on long enough to produce some useful guidance for people, like so many in the complexity of health service, who bring other people together to make something different happen. This is a game any number can play. Here, for starters, are a few pointers from my own experience:

If nobody can be effectively in general charge, everyone associated with a collective activity is partly in charge of it—and should act accordingly. Thus, every participant is, *to some self-selected degree*, a leader. How big a part each person plays depends on how responsible that person feels for the general outcome of the collective effort.

Clarence Pearson and Gary Filerman, in their "Looking Ahead" chapter of the *Critical Issues* book (2001), highlighted some of the special challenges that await what they call the "transformational leader" in global health. It takes an unusual measure of both self-confidence and tact for such a person to use his or her "breadth of experience" to muscle into the policy domains of more conventional colleagues.

Transformation arrived at by suasion and compromise makes for fuzzy boundaries, interim outcomes, and ambiguous arrangements. Explaining these to coworkers and constituents, who may have learned to honor and obey the comfortable clarity of narrower disciplines, may turn out to be even harder than arriving at them. A wider outlook never seems to be the path to instant popularity.

Just a few more observations about the special chemistry of a nobody-in-charge system: Do not try to draw it on an organizational chart. Rigid two-dimensional lines and boxes will distort the reality you want to achieve—one that is actually much more akin to chemical reactions in a liquid solution.

Looser is, in practice, usually better. The fewer and narrower are the "rules" that everyone involved must follow, the more room there is for individual discretion and initiative, small-group insights and inventions, regional adaptations, and functional differences. Flexibility and informality are good for coworkers' morale, constituency support, investor enthusiasm, and customer satisfaction.

In such a system, planning is not "architecture": it is more like "fluid drive." Real-life planning is improvisation on a general sense of direction—announced by the few, perhaps, but only after genuine consultation with the many who will need to improvise on it.

And if we are all going to be partly in charge, then information is for sharing, not hoarding. Planning staffs, systems analysis units, and others whose full-time assignment is to think, should not report only in secret to some "boss." Their relevant knowledge has to be shared with all those who might be able to use it to advance the organization's purpose.

You will remember that, some years ago, Japanese auto companies, advised by a genius engineer from Michigan, started sharing much more information on productivity with workers on their assembly lines. It was small groups of workers on the factory floor, reacting to that information, who thought up the myriad little changes that increased speed, cut costs, improved quality, and enhanced productivity. Quite suddenly, Japanese automobiles became globally supercompetitive.

Attitudes for Leaders

Because the demand for leaders keeps growing faster than the demand for even the hottest specialists, many specialized professionals nowadays find themselves drawn to spend at least part of their time and energy as generalist leaders. This seems to be especially the case in the health services—because they are mostly a service, not a production, activity; because the range of knowledge required is so broad that no one can "know it all"; and because health service professionals are ultimately concerned with the minds and bodies of individuals, each somewhat different from all the others.

A quarter-century ago, Peter Drucker (1980, p. 208) wrote wisely about the transition from professional to generalist. The professional, he said, "does not cease to be a 'professional'; he must not cease to be one. But he acquires an additional dimension of understanding, additional vision, and the sense of responsibility for the survival and importance of the whole that distinguishes the manager from the subordinate and the citizen from the subject."

Back when a book called *The One Minute Manager* hit the best-seller lists, I tried to compress in a short article what I had learned, from experience and from study, about the "generalist mindset" for leadership. My tongue was only half in cheek. There had to be a market niche for a learning tool that leaders, who are usually in a hurry, could absorb on the run.

For the generalist leader, I reasoned, the steepest part of the learning curve is not skills but attitudes. Those of us who presume to take the lead in a democracy, where nobody is even supposed to be in charge, seem to need an arsenal of eight attitudes (reading time: one minute) indispensable to the management of complexity:

- First, a lively intellectual curiosity, an interest in everything—because everything really is related to everything else—and, therefore, to what you are doing, whatever that is.

- Second, a genuine interest in what other people think and why they think that way, which means for a start that you have to be at peace with yourself.

- Third, a feeling of special responsibility to envision a future that is different from a straight-line projection of the present. Trends are not destiny.

- Fourth, a hunch that most risks are there not to be avoided but to be taken.

- Fifth, a mind-set that crises are normal, tensions can be promising, and complexity is fun.

- Sixth, a realization that paranoia and self-pity are reserved for people who *do not* want to be leaders.

- Seventh, a sense of *personal* responsibility for the *general* outcome of your efforts.

- Eighth, a quality I call "unwarranted optimism": the conviction that there must be some more upbeat outcome than would result from adding up all the available expert advice.

References

Cleveland, H. "Introduction: Toward an International Poverty Line." In J. McHale and M. C. McHale (eds.), *Basic Human Needs: A Framework for Action*. New Brunswick, N.J.: Transaction Books, 1978.

Cleveland, H. *The Knowledge Executive: Leadership in an Information Society*. New York: Talley/Dutton, 1985.

Cleveland, H. *The Information Imperative Embraces Liberté, Egalité, and Access*. Boston: World Times, 1997.

Cleveland, H. *Nobody in Charge: Essays on the Future of Leadership*. San Francisco: Jossey-Bass, 2002.

Daulaire, N. "The Nonprofit Sector in Partnership with Government." In C. E. Koop, C. E. Pearson, and M. R. Schwarz (eds.), *Critical Issues in Global Health*. Foreword by J. Carter. San Francisco: Jossey-Bass, 2002, pp. 423–429.

Drucker, P. *Managing in Turbulent Times*. New York: Harper & Row, 1980.

Foege, W. H. "Infectious Diseases." In C. E. Koop, C. E. Pearson, and M. R. Schwarz (eds.), *Critical Issues in Global Health*. Foreword by J. Carter. San Francisco: Jossey-Bass, 2002, pp. 111–116.

"Human Genome Survey: Ingenious Medicine." *The Economist*, June 29, 2000.

Koop, C. E., Pearson, C. E., and Schwartz, M. R. (eds.). *Critical Issues in Global Health*. Foreword by J. Carter. San Francisco: Jossey-Bass, 2002.

McHale, J., and McHale, M. C. *Basic Human Needs: A Framework for Action*. Foreword by M. Tolba. Introduction by H. Cleveland. New Brunswick, N.J.: Transaction Books, 1978.

Naidoo, K. "The Role of the Nonprofit Sector." In C. E. Koop, C. E. Pearson, and M. R. Schwarz (eds.), *Critical Issues in Global Health*. Foreword by J. Carter. San Francisco: Jossey-Bass, 2002, pp. 406–413.

Pearson, C., and Filerman, G. "Looking Ahead." In C. E. Koop, C. E. Pearson, and M. R. Schwarz (eds.), *Critical Issues in Global Health*. Foreword by J. Carter. San Francisco: Jossey-Bass, 2002.

Ramalingaswami, V. "India." In C. E. Koop, C. E. Pearson, and M. R. Schwarz (eds.), *Critical Issues in Global Health*. Foreword by J. Carter. San Francisco: Jossey-Bass, 2002, pp. 62–70.

United Nations. "Universal Declaration of Human Rights." *Yearbook of the United Nations, 1948–1949*. Lake Success, N.Y.: United Nations, 1950.

6

HIV/AIDS

Lessons from Brazil

Susan Dentzer

When the definitive history is written about the world's response to the HIV/AIDS (human immunodeficiency virus–acquired immunodeficiency syndrome) pandemic, a number of developments will surely loom large. Among them will be the growing realization during the 1980s that, short of the development of an effective vaccine, preventing HIV's spread would prove staggeringly difficult. Also notable was the relatively rapid development of antiretroviral drugs and, by the mid-1990s, the demonstrable success of combination-drug therapy in postponing the progression of disease. Not long after came the recognition that treatment and prevention must go hand in hand—because, without treatment, infected persons had no reason to seek medical care, where they in turn could be counseled on how to avoid infecting others. Then came the shocking awareness that, with the exception of patients in the richest nations, treatment was mostly out of reach for most of the world because of the prohibitively high prices of antiretroviral drugs (ARVs).

Although these realities emerged across many countries and continents, perhaps one single country grasped them most completely and soonest: Brazil. The story of how this South American nation of 175 million rose to meet its HIV/AIDS challenge has been one of the few bright lights in a mostly grim global picture. In the 1990s, Brazil was one of the first countries to provide free HIV/AIDS treatment with ARVs to its population of infected patients. It was also among the first countries to openly challenge global pharmaceutical companies to cut ARV prices, warning that Brazil would otherwise manufacture its own generic copies (several of which it subsequently did). Brazil has also launched arguably the boldest public health campaign worldwide, adopting needle-exchange programs for intravenous-drug users and rejecting abstinence as a prevention strategy in favor of encouraging widespread condom use. In this aspect in particular, Brazil's AIDS-prevention policies represent a marked departure from other countries, including the United States.

In the opinion of most global health experts, these approaches have paid off handsomely. In the mid-1990s, the World Bank projected that 1.2 million Brazilians would be infected with HIV by 2000. Today, however, the number of those estimated to be infected with the virus is half that amount. The seroprevalence rate among those aged fifteen to forty-nine years is 0.65 percent, sharply below the 5 percent seroprevalence rate in Uganda, for example, or the 20 percent rate in South Africa, the country with the single greatest number of people infected with HIV. In 2003, the Brazilian government was awarded the prestigious Gates Award in Global Health by the Bill and Melinda Gates Foundation for being "a model for combating HIV/AIDS in developing countries." The Brazilian government promised to use the U.S.$1 million in prize money to fund community-based AIDS groups caring for orphans and people living with HIV/AIDS.

"Social statistics are human beings with the tears washed away," the saying goes. One relevant statistic is that roughly 135,000 Brazilians now have access to antiretroviral therapy, provided free by the national government. One of those human beings who make up the statistic is Gloria Pinheiro. A woman in her late forties who appears much older, Pinheiro lives just across the bay from Rio de Janeiro in the town of Sao Goncalo, in a home that is really an unfinished construction site. I met her there in 2003 on a reporting trip to Brazil (under the auspices of my employer, *The NewsHour with Jim Lehrer* on PBS, and the *NewsHour*'s partner, the Henry J. Kaiser Family Foundation). Pinheiro told me that her late husband, Marco, was in the process of building the home when he died in 2000, one month after being diagnosed with AIDS. He had told her that he had acquired the disease through surgery. She told me she trusted her husband, who had told her he was faithful to her. But she acknowledged that, since his death, she had also learned that he had frequented prostitutes. Soon after her husband's death, Pinheiro discovered that she, too, was infected with HIV. When I met her she had been actively under care for several years at a local public health clinic and on ARV therapy as well.

Through a translator, Pinheiro told me: "I depend on the medicines that the Brazilian government gives me, and like most of the people with HIV, we're very poor people. We wouldn't be able to survive without that. If we can't even afford food, there is no way we would be able to afford the medication. Imagine us paying for medication."

In a country with a gross domestic product (GDP) per capita of about $7,600 in 2003—measured in purchasing-power parity terms, that is about one-fifth the per capita income of the United States—asking peasants like Pinheiro to pay for medication was clearly out of the question. But at the same time, to Brazilians, so was consigning tens of thousands of HIV-infected persons to premature deaths over a small matter like the prohibitive cost of pharmaceuticals. The policies that evolved from these realizations have since saved or prolonged the lives of tens of thousands, including Gloria Pinheiro.

There is no doubt that Brazil had a number of distinct advantages over other developing countries facing HIV/AIDS. For one thing, it had far more in the way of financial resources to bring to the problem than most—because technically it is a middle-income country, with a per capita GDP about six times that of Uganda. AIDS also came along in Brazil at a unique time in the country's history, when democracy was about to be restored after decades of military rule. For all the reasons that make Brazil a singular case, however, its story is well worth capturing. When the world one day looks back on the HIV pandemic, it will be evident that at least a few countries and their citizens did the right thing.

Brazil's Response to HIV/AIDS

The seeds of Brazil's HIV/AIDS response were sown in the mid-1980s, just as a large number of AIDS patients were first turning up in urban hospitals and clinics. After two decades of military rule ended in 1985, the country was democratizing with the election of a civilian president. A new Brazilian constitution was adopted, guaranteeing among other things freedom of speech and the right to health care. As a result, a variety of new social movements and organizations were taking root—and feeling newly empowered to speak out on issues like the rights of women and gays and improvements in health care.

It was only a few years earlier, in 1982, that Brazil had become aware of its first known instance of AIDS. In 1983, more cases followed, almost all of them involving gay and bisexual men. Gay rights groups began to press local governments in states like Sao Paolo to institute special clinic-based programs for AIDS patients. At the time, these were mainly focused on treating patients' opportunistic infections because little else was available. In 1986 came the founding of ABIA (Associação Brasileira Interdisciplinar de AIDS, a nongovernmental organization (NGO) created to monitor and advocate for public policies on HIV and AIDS.

ABIA's current president, Cristina Pimenta, told me in a 2003 interview that her organization and other NGOs quickly came to play a critical role as liaisons between government and the then-marginalized population groups most affected by HIV. Among other victories, ABIA helped to persuade the government to enact legislation barring discrimination against those infected with the virus.

In pressing for action against HIV and AIDS, the organization by default also assumed a broader role in advocating for the entire health of the Brazilian population. One example: helping to persuade the national government to regulate private blood banks to require HIV screening of the blood supply.

"This dialogue with the government of Brazil was not always so easy," Pimenta told me in an interview. Although there was often agreement among NGOs and the government on needs and objectives, there were substantial disagreements as to how quickly measures needed to be implemented. "But the social movement was saying that people were dying, and the population was becoming more and more infected," Pimenta said. And over time, the connections forged among NGOs and the government resulted in measures that took far longer in other countries or were never enacted at all.

In Pimenta's view, a key reason for the success of ABIA and other NGOs working in HIV/AIDS was that they were born out of the broader citizenship and democratization movements. As a result, in Brazil, making progress against the disease was seen almost from the start as not being a fringe issue but as part of the essence of the new Brazilian democracy. Similarly, the provision of services to persons with HIV was equated with preserving the rights guaranteed to them under the constitution—rights not only to state-provided health care but also to lives of dignity as human beings.

In Brazil, as elsewhere, all health care is local—or at least, it begins that way. In terms of the provision of services, health departments in Brazil's thirteen states and their largest municipalities were the first to mobilize to provide care for AIDS patients. In the early 1980s, an energetic physician named Paolo Teixeira was heading the health department in the large and prosperous state of Sao Paolo, where Brazil's first AIDS cases were recognized. (He has since gone on to head the Brazilian national AIDS and sexually transmitted diseases program and, subsequently, the World Health Organization [WHO] HIV/AIDS program.) I interviewed Teixeira in

2003 while he was still heading the national program and on the eve of his departure for WHO in Geneva.

Teixeira had taken the lead on coordinating Sao Paolo's response as soon as it became clear that an epidemic was developing in the state. Then, as cases began to appear in other states, he and other Sao Paolo officials were called in as consultants to help them devise their own programs. Finally, after thirteen of Brazil's twenty-six states had enacted programs, it became clear that an overarching national effort was also needed, so the Ministry of Health created a program to focus on HIV and other sexually transmitted diseases. The ministry and the national AIDS program negotiated a loan from the World Bank to launch various treatment and prevention efforts. In 1992, discussions were launched with the bank for a second round of assistance.

By this point, AIDS had spread beyond the homosexual population to intravenous-drug users, many of whom were heterosexual. As a result, a growing number of infected women who were partners of drug users began to show up in local AIDS clinics. I met one such woman at Sao Paolo's Emilio Ribas hospital in 2003—Rosana Bento Teixeira (no relation to Paolo Teixeira), a woman in her thirties. She told me she had contracted HIV from her first husband, an intravenous-drug user, whom she had divorced some years earlier and who had died before she learned she was infected. She was remarried and had had a son with her new husband before she fell ill with AIDS.

Through channels such as this, a major outbreak of the virus into the general heterosexual population of Brazil seemed a distinct possibility. In 1993, with the second World Bank package still under discussion, consultants from the bank issued their dire forecast that 1.2 million Brazilians would become infected by 2000.

Brazilian officials believed their best hope of stemming such an outbreak called for drastic prevention measures. As a result, so-called harm reduction programs for intravenous-drug users, including free needle exchanges, were put in place in large and populous cities like

Rio and Sao Paolo and then elsewhere throughout the country. That was in sharp contrast to the thrust of policy in the United States, for example, where needle-exchange programs were widely viewed as fostering illegal drug use and where Congress has prohibited any federal expenditures on such programs since 1998.

For the vast non-intravenous-drug-using portion of Brazil's population, effective prevention programs were clearly going to have to deal with the subject of sex. Some Brazilian AIDS experts assert that there were some short-lived programs aimed at stressing abstinence. That had been the case in Uganda, where a government-backed prevention program built around ABC—abstinence, being faithful, or using condoms—had made decisive inroads into slowing the HIV infection rate. But while reporting in Brazil, I never found any solid evidence that programs stressing abstinence had ever been taken seriously. Artur Kalichman, coordinator of the state of Sao Paolo's AIDS and sexually transmitted disease program, told me that encouraging abstinence was simply ineffective as a strategy for dealing with the broad public. "Abstinence could be an individual choice," he said. "And it's very respectable. I cannot disagree with somebody who decides to be abstinent; it's okay for sure. And it works. But as a public health message, I don't believe that it's feasible, and I don't believe that it works. Not ideologically, [but] based on evidence data available all over the world."

With views like Kalichman's constituting the prevailing Brazilian public health perspective, a major push was launched to encourage the use of condoms. The national government began to purchase and give away for free millions of condoms a year, even to the point of installing condom-dispensing units in government offices in the capital city, Brasilia. In 2003, officials told me that the government would buy and give away for free nearly four hundred million condoms that year and to triple that number over the next three years. Discussions were under way about investing in a condom factory to make that possible. Although the standard male condom has been most widely promoted, Brazil has also become the only

national government to date to buy and distribute the female condom as well.

At state, local, and national expense, free condoms of both types
have been given out to many of the nation's prostitutes. (The sale
of sexual favors by one person to another is legal in Brazil; only
operation of a brothel is illegal.) To accomplish that, the national
AIDS and sexually transmitted disease program has worked closely
with various NGOs—the likes of which it is hard to imagine taking root in the United States. One, called Prostitution Civil Rights
and Health, is run by Gabriela Silva Leite, a retired prostitute from
Rio de Janeiro. Although acknowledging that there had hardly been
a controlled study to prove the theory, Leite told me that the HIV
infection rate of 6 percent among Brazil's 170,000 prostitutes would
easily have been sharply higher without the free condom program.

To alert the general population of the risks of HIV/AIDS, the
national AIDS program also oversaw the launch of a massive print
and television advertising campaign that also focused on encouraging condom use. These tended to overtly portray sexuality and
sexual encounters among heterosexuals and homosexuals alike.
In 2003, I watched a collection of commercials paid for by the
National AIDS and sexually transmitted disease program and concluded that, stripped of their warnings about the use of condoms,
some could be mistaken for pornography.

I told Teixeira that if U.S. Health and Human Services Secretary Tommy Thompson had his department pay to develop such
commercials, he would be fired approximately five minutes after the
first one aired. Texeira laughed. "The Brazilian culture is more tol-
erant in talking about sex and sex behavior" than that of countries
like the United States, he observed with considerable understate-
ment. As a result, the heavy promotion of condoms "is not considered aggressive by people in general." Teixeira acknowledged that,
in a nation where four out of five adults describe themselves as
Roman Catholics, church authorities had sometimes protested. I
later asked Humberto da Costa, Brazil's Health Minister, about

those protests. He shrugged. "We say to religi[ous] groups, 'Okay, you have your idea, but we are only thinking about health. For this reason we respect your opinion, but we are going this way, telling the people to use condoms, telling the people to practice safe sex, and I think this is the best way.'"

There is little doubt that these prevention efforts have paid off. Kalichman told me in 2003 that new infections have leveled off among gay men and have fallen among intravenous-drug users. At the same time, there was scarcely any reason to declare victory against the spread of HIV. As of today, infection rates are still rising among women. In the 1980s, Kalichman told me, the ratio of infected Brazilian men to infected women was 20 to 1; as of 2003, he said, it was 2 to 1, and as low as 1 to 1 for asymptomatic patients with HIV. "Nowadays, not only [in] Sao Paolo but in Brazil as a whole, what is on the rise is heterosexual transmission," he said. The virus is also spreading beyond the major cities like Sao Paolo and Rio to smaller and medium-sized cities, especially in the interior of the country and the northeast. An equally worrisome trend is a rise in new infections among prison inmates, which World Bank representatives in particular have pressed Brazil to address.

What can never be known, of course, is how much worse any of these trends would have been had Brazil not adopted its prevention strategies. Equally uncertain is how prevention would have fared had it not been coupled with arguably even more aggressive strategies on treatment. And it is in the treatment realm in particular that Brazil made what is probably its most significant and lasting contribution to the global response to HIV/AIDS.

Government-Sponsored Treatment of HIV/AIDS

By the mid-1980s, largely under pressure from AIDS activists in the United States, the U.S. government and major pharmaceutical companies had launched major efforts to research and develop anti-AIDS drugs. The first drug that turned out to be effective specifically against the properties of HIV, a retrovirus, was zidovudine, or AZT. Originally developed as a cancer therapy, it showed the ability to block an enzyme central to the process by which HIV replicated itself in the body. Soon other early-generation ARVs came on the market as well.

These developments did not go unnoticed in Brazil, where in 1991 the national government determined that ARVs should be available to all HIV-positive people who needed them. The government began purchasing and distributing AZT through clinics nationwide. In effect, a deal was struck whereby the national government would pay for the costly ARVs and state and local governments bore the costs of other drugs, such as antibiotics to fight opportunistic infections. Ironically, in some poorer localities, that often meant that patients got the ARVs provided by the national government but did not get antibiotics from nearly destitute local clinics. In Sao Goncalo, the poor town across the bay from Rio where I met Pinheiro, AIDS patients and activists ultimately had gone to court and won a judge's ruling ordering the locality to boost services and provide the drugs.

In 1996, a Brazilian delegation traveled to Vancouver, Canada, where that year's biannual International AIDS Conference took place. Among the breakthrough findings reported at the conference was evidence that combinations of several ARV drugs—so-called triple therapy—dramatically lowered levels of HIV in the blood of infected patients. Teixeira told me that he and other officials quickly did the obvious math: at a minimum, their outlays for ARVs would triple. "And the conclusion was that it would be absolutely impossible to [carry out] this policy by buying drugs from big companies and paying the prices" they charged, Teixeira said.

He and other Brazilian officials turned to experts at the Oswaldo Cruz Foundation, located on a leafy campus in Rio de Janeiro. Generally known by an acronym, *Fiocruz*, it is a quasi-governmental private foundation that is in many respects Brazil's equivalent of a cross between the National Institutes of Health and the Food and Drug

Administration. Fiocruz also has a research, development, and manufacturing arm called Far Manguinhos that had long focused on developing drugs and vaccines to fight Brazil's tropical diseases. In 1997, the production plant at Far Manguinhos began making copies of some ARVs that had either gone off patent or had never been patented in Brazil. As a result, Teixeira told me, Brazil's costs for those medications plummeted by 85 percent.

Within a year or two, as new ARVs came on the market and new combination therapies proved effective, Teixeira and other officials realized that Brazil also needed access to drugs that were still under patent protection. In the United States, retail prices for these newer triple therapies were running U.S.$10,000 and up per year. Brazilian officials approached several manufacturers, such as Merck and Company, Inc., and offered to negotiate price reductions. If such price cuts were not forthcoming, they warned, Brazil would begin manufacturing the drugs itself under so-called compulsory licenses—and under provisions of global trade law that allowed it to do so to meet local public health emergencies.

To buttress the threat, Brazilian officials gave the companies samples of equivalent versions of their drugs that researchers at Far Manguinhos had already produced. By the time I visited in 2003, Far Manguinhos was producing six ARVs and had developed the capability to make an additional six more. Jorges Lima de Magalhaes, production manager at Far Manguinhos, told me that the companies were stunned. "I do think they were surprised when they saw a developing country like Brazil producing these drugs and the fact that it was being used in a socially responsible way. In other words, it wasn't for profit, it was to meet the needs of the Brazilian people and the people sick with AIDS."

The homemade generic copies of on-patent drugs clearly succeeded in getting the pharmaceutical companies' attention. The Brazilians were "very canny negotiators," an official of one major global pharmaceutical company told me in a conversation on background in 2003. "They played to win." Most of the pharmaceutical companies gave in and agreed to cut prices by a range of 45 to 70 percent per drug, according to Teixeira's calculations. The price cuts enabled Brazil to maintain its policy of providing free ARVs to tens of thousands of patients who met specific criteria for HIV viral load and other indicators.

The resulting payoff was enormous. After five years of providing free combination therapy, average nationwide mortality from AIDS had fallen about 50 percent. In some major cities, the decrease was as high as 70 percent. In total, the national government estimated that eighty thousand lives had been saved.

In addition, the strategy of providing free ARVs turned out to be surprisingly cost-effective. With patients staying well longer, the rate of hospitalization among HIV-infected patients plummeted. So did unemployment and premature retirement among those with HIV. Within five years, Brazil had saved about U.S.$2.2 billion in hospital costs, money that it was able to plow back into other aspects of its HIV program.

In a broader context, Brazil's actions over this period also played a key role in pushing down ARV prices worldwide. From 2000 to 2003, the lowest prices available worldwide for on-patent ARVs fell by a factor of ten. There were, of course, forces other than Brazilian pressure pushing down prices during this time. In the 1990s, Indian drug manufacturers like Cipla had also developed generic versions of ARVs that they offered developing countries for less than $100 per patient per year. In addition to prompting pharmaceutical companies to cut prices, these forces combined to prompt massive revisions of the companies' pricing policies. Merck, for example, in March 2001 adopted a three-tiered global pricing policy. The policy took into account both national income and HIV seroprevalence in a given country, with the result that most of the nations hardest hit by HIV would be charged drastically less for ARVs than prices for the same drugs in wealthy countries like the United States.

But beyond what Brazil helped to accomplish in price cuts, the country's actions also left behind important lessons on other fronts.

To distribute ARVs free to patients around the country, it developed a computerized system installed at clinics around the country to keep track of which drugs were dispensed, to what patient, and when. The system was thought to have been helpful in several respects. For one thing, it drastically cut down on opportunities for corruption. Teixeira told me in 2003 that there had been reports of some HIV patients selling the drugs after they had obtained them free from clinics, presumably for export to other countries. The government had launched investigations and legal proceedings against some patients, but on balance, government officials believed the tracking system had succeeded in keeping such corruption to a minimum.

Even more important, the computerized tracking system had helped to clear up an important question: Could Brazilian patients adhere to the arduous ARV treatment regimen? For years there had been doubt in some quarters that patients in developing countries could maintain the then-rigorous regimen of triple-dose therapy, which sometimes required taking as many as several dozen pills a day on a set schedule. It was no idle question. Patients who did not take their drugs obviously risked their own lives because many who stopped taking medication would experience steep rises in viral load and susceptibility to AIDS-related infections. Nonadherence could also hasten the process of developing drug-resistant strains of HIV— a process that had already become evident around the world with the earliest generation of ARVs.

But with the computerized tracking system, a Brazilian clinic dispensing the pills had an important tool for monitoring adherence: it could keep track of whether patients were coming in on schedule to pick up their monthly doses of medications. Patients I met while in Brazil told me their clinics and physicians had been proactive in staying in touch with them to make sure they were adhering to treatment regimens. Although no rigorous studies have been done comparing patient adherence in Brazil versus that in the United States, for example, from comparisons across small studies, it appears that Brazil has no worse a problem with adherence than the United States or the United Kingdom.

When I visited Far Manguinhos in 2003, production manager Lima de Magalhaes told me that researchers there were continuing to develop copies of the newest ARVs coming onto the market. One example was Fuseon, a GlaxoSmithKline drug that was running U.S.$20,000 a year in the United States and that Brazilians had satisfied themselves they could copy. "We have the technologies to continue in pace with whatever is being produced," Lima de Magalhaes said. And as before, Brazilian officials told me they would continue the strategy of asking manufacturers first for price cuts—but backing up the request with the threat of being able to produce the drugs if manufacturers did not give in.

A major worry among pharmaceutical companies was whether Brazil would ever go a step farther than this—and, like the Indian companies, begin making generic copies of on-patent drugs for export to other countries. When I asked Health Minister Da Costa about this prospect, he insisted that it was not in the cards. "We want to negotiate the prices," he said. "We are in a position to produce many of them, but we want to negotiate." He did say, however, that Brazil would continue its policy of helping other countries with "technology transfer"—that is, showing them how they, too, could make the drugs if the need arose. And in fact, Brazil had begun showing a handful of countries, such as other Portuguese-speaking nations like Mozambique and Angola, how they might be able to manufacture the drugs if the need arose.

I discussed this issue further with Rosemeire Munhoz, who until late 2003 headed the External Cooperation Department of Brazil's national AIDS program. (Like Teixeira, she was eventually recruited away—in her case, by UNAIDS, the United Nations' umbrella AIDS agency—to help implement HIV/AIDS strategies at the global level.) Munhoz said the notion of getting drugs or drug-manufacturing technology into the hands of poorer countries "is really a very big issue globally when we think about the control of AIDS internationally. We think that we have to reduce the gap existing between the developed countries and developing countries, and we think that is a kind of human right to have for all of the people coming from developed countries or developing countries to have access to antiretroviral medicine."

In addition to showing other countries how they might make medicines, Munhoz and other Brazilian officials told me they were keen to show other countries how to create systems to administer the drugs and monitor adherence, much as Brazil had. They also wanted to help school other nations in the notion that treatment and prevention were inseparable—for example, that intravenous-drug users sick with AIDS were more likely to participate in needle-exchange programs if they also knew that ARVs were available to extend their lives.

It is not "like *Sophie's Choice*, that movie," Sao Paolo's Kalichman told me. By that, he meant that there was no realistic option that developing countries in the midst of the AIDS pandemic should content themselves with low-cost prevention strategies and not expect the world to offer assistance in providing treatment. Treatment and prevention, he said, "are synergic. The one benefits the other, and [the result is] better outcomes in both." In this sense, he said, Brazil is "an example. I mean, if we can do it here, why can't people do it in other places? Not necessarily in the way we are doing it, the same way, because the reality may be very different from Brazil in other countries. But we are more than a model. I think we are a reference, or an example that things can be done."

Future of the Brazilian Approach

When I left Brazil in May 2003, Kalichman's notion of Brazil as an example for the rest of the world to follow was much in the air. Like star hitters on a baseball farm team, Teixeira and Munhoz were about to be recruited to bring their expertise to the global HIV "big leagues"—he to WHO and she to UNAIDS. Teixeira and Health

Minister Da Costa were soon to travel to Washington to accept the Gates Award at the annual gala dinner of the Global Health Council, the international organization that selects each year's Gates Award winner. When Teixeira and Da Costa walked onto the stage to accept the award, the crowd greeted them with a standing ovation and cheers. There was an ineffable sense that, after nearly two decades of unrelenting bad news in the HIV pandemic, a corner had been turned, at least somewhere.

In the global health community, there was much loose talk about the Brazilian "model"—as if the country's HIV response, built up over two decades, could simply be purchased off the shelf and put in place elsewhere. Some accused Teixeira of fostering such talk by actually using the word "model" from time to time. Others, like Pimenta of ABIA, were more cautious. "I like to refer not to the Brazilian model, but the Brazilian response, because I think it's a combination of actions and of policies, of resources that were allocated. It's not a model, because a model is something that you can take somewhere and copy it, and you can't copy a response. You can learn from it, and there are lessons to be learned from Brazil: the commitment of the government, the partnership between the civil movement and nongovernmental organizations with the government. You can look and see that you had good results, what were the strategies that worked. So there are lessons to be learned."

And there will surely be more lessons to learn from Brazil because, like most countries in the midst of the HIV pandemic, it is hardly out of the woods. In the slums, or *favelas*, of Rio or Sao Paolo, thousands are still becoming infected with HIV. Statistics clearly show that more and more are women and, increasingly, desperately poor. In a grim demonstration of the epidemic coming full circle, the country has now seen its first instances of second-generation maternal-to-child transmission of HIV, as babies who were born with HIV grow up and become mothers themselves. The new leftist government of President Luiz Inacio Lula da Silva (known as "Lula") seems thoroughly committed to carrying on the fight against HIV. But even so, AIDS activists like Pimenta worry about maintaining financial support for prevention strategies that must be continuous over a long period.

Still, across the bay from Rio, there is Pinheiro—one of the more than six hundred thousand HIV-infected Brazilians who are arguably still alive today because their government and their fellow citizens intervened. When I last saw Pinheiro, it was early on a spring evening, after we had spent part of an afternoon talking about her battle with AIDS. The dusk was settling, and the lights of Rio were beginning to twinkle across the bay. Pinheiro had just finished taking several pills, the latest installments of her multidrug AIDS cocktails. She was lying on the couch in her living room, beneath a portrait of Jesus, resting as she often did after downing the medication. One of her two grown daughters was close by. Together they were engaged in their regular nighttime ritual: the grown daughter in her twenties teaching her forty-six-year-old mother, a child of Brazil's worst slums, to read. The day's text was a pamphlet from the Ministry of Health on preventing HIV.

Reference

Proceedings of the XI International Conference on AIDS. Vancouver, Canada, July 7–12, 1996.

7

• •

Corruption and Health Care
Need for New Solutions

Peter Eigen

Like disease, corruption is the enemy of the poor and the vulnerable. Countless lives are lost every day when corrupt officials intercept vital medicines and healthier supplies destined to meet those suffering from diseases such as HIV/AIDS (human immunodeficiency virus–acquired immunodeficiency syndrome), malaria, or tuberculosis. When corruption prevents the supply of medicines—or undermines the delivery of basic health care services—the consequences can be devastating.

Disease of Corruption

In the city of Bangalore in southern India, an independent survey of the quality of maternity health services for the urban poor conducted in 2000 by the nongovernmental organization (NGO) Public Affairs Center (Web site: http://www.pacindia.org/Programmes_Activities/02Research) revealed that the poor pay huge amounts of extortion money in their interactions with the public maternity hospitals. The average patient in a maternity ward run by the city corporation pays 1,089 rupees (about U.S.$22) in bribes to receive adequate medical care. Furthermore, 61 percent of the respondents were forced to pay for medicines, although public policy clearly mandates that they be given free of charge.

The corruption challenge in the global health sector is complex. It extends from the petty corruption that robs the poor of basic treatment to the deeply ingrained collusion and corrupt dealings that threaten the entire health framework. In terms of the latter, it is necessary to examine the role of the pharmaceutical companies that make cures to global health crises possible.

In John Le Carré's recent novel *The Constant Gardener* (2001) the reader is led through a labyrinth of intrigue and corporate deception, of stark choices whose consequences are a matter of life and death. The kernel of Le Carré's story is corruption, and the protagonists in his tale grapple with the competing interests of short-term corporate profit and a population desperately fending off the effects of a fatal epidemic.

At Transparency International (TI), the leading global NGO engaged in the fight against corruption, our national chapters live in, and report back from, the factual equivalent of this twilight world, in which individual, corporate, and government interests collectively lay waste to entire societies in their desire for enrichment. Corruption is an institutional disease: it spreads through the body politic with amazing rapidity and has proved remarkably resistant to cure.

Unhealthy World Order?

In terms of corruption, the pharmaceutical industry is at great risk. Corruption threatens research and its publication, the drug-licensing process, marketing efforts, and indeed, delivery and distribution in some parts of the world. These risks have a knock-on effect throughout the health care "chain."

A few unscrupulous companies could undermine the whole health care industry, a sector whose reputation is all-important. If those who seek to save the lives of others are undermined by a few rotten apples, the whole profession suffers. This is particularly acute in the case of physicians who prescribe drugs to patients who put their trust in the medical expertise and judgment of physicians. Annual spending on health care in the United States alone amounts to more than U.S.$1 trillion, and in many developed countries, where the bill goes to the insurance company, health care is open to fraud and abuse as an industry where the client is not billed directly and cannot check line by line the description of services rendered. Again, the rotten few undermine the dedication of the many.

TI's Bribe Payers' Survey 2002 (http://www.transparency.org/surveys/index.html#bpi) looks at the supply side of bribery. It shows the propensity of companies from various countries to pay bribes when operating in other countries than their own—and also which sectors are most perceived as likely to pay such bribes. The pharmaceutical and medical care industries come in the middle of the rankings, with a score of 4.3 out of a perfect 10. This is a better result than in the construction and arms industries but worse than in forestry and banking.

In December 2002, Syncor International Corporation and its subsidiary Syncor Taiwan were charged by the U.S. Securities and Exchange Commission and the U.S. Department of Justice with having made illegal payments to physicians in Taiwan, Mexico, Belgium, Luxembourg, and France through practices such as inflated invoicing, payment of improper commissions for referrals, and direct gifts to physicians and state hospitals to ensure that they continued to order Syncor pharmaceutical supplies.

Such schemes bypassed internal accounting controls. The good news is that Syncor voluntarily disclosed the allegations, and substantial fines were paid by the company and its Taiwan subsidiary. But this cannot be dismissed as an isolated incident.

In February 2003, Italian prosecutors began investigations into GlaxoSmithKline for allegedly bribing physicians to prescribe the company's drugs. The bribes apparently ranged from holidays in the Caribbean to hi-fi systems. In 2002, the same company faced allegations in Germany that physicians were offered free trips to

World Cup football and Formula One racing. As of May 2004, the investigations continued, with as many as four thousand physicians implicated in shady practices that, if confirmed, undermine the integrity of health care systems.

The corruption that Le Carré was writing about was also in the pharmaceutical industry, but it was set against a background of state violence in Moi's Kenya. The lessons are clear. Corruption in the health sector is a particular threat in strong states where the judiciary lacks independence and where other government organs responsible for assuring probity in health procurement and delivery cannot provide a counterweight to those who want deals done, including in their own interest. Weak or even failing states—many burdened with public health crises and poverty—are vulnerable to corruption and to suffering more corruption than others.

Building National Integrity Systems

What role can civil society play in cleaning up global health care systems? TI's own mission is "to curb corruption by mobilizing a global coalition to promote and strengthen international and national integrity systems." Although the basic concepts and foundations of an integrity system need to be clearly understood, including their relevance to health care as a public good, it is equally important that the resulting solutions be grounded in reality and practicality.

TI has adopted a National Integrity System (NIS) approach as its core lens for analysis of transparency. The NIS approach unlocks a new form of diagnosis and potential cure for corruption. Instead of looking at separate institutions (such as the judiciary) or separate rules and practices (such as criminal law) and then focusing on stand-alone reform programs, it looks at interrelationships, interdependence, and the combined effectiveness in a holistic approach.

Many anticorruption strategies have failed because they have been too narrowly focused. The pillars on which an NIS rest are, therefore, all those institutions and practices that work together to protect society against corruption. If the system is wholly dependent on a single "pillar," such as a "benign dictator," for example, or only a few functioning pillars, it will be vulnerable to collapse. Solutions to corruption must relate to the other parts of the overall system.

Establishing a sound NIS also requires a move away from top-down reforms. Instead, the system should emphasize "horizontal accountability," where power is dispersed, where no single actor has a monopoly, and where each one is separately accountable. It also requires the systematic identification of gaps and weaknesses and also opportunities for strengthening or augmenting each of these pillars into a coherent framework. Any effort to bolster the health sector against corruption, for instance, requires cooperation across pillars, from the private sector driving the medical research to the budgeting process for health care–related issues to the medical practitioners themselves, as part of the health care delivery apparatus.

The solution advocated by TI to fight corruption is to foster, evaluate, and strengthen NISs in line with local conditions. So TI's approach to successful anticorruption strategies hinges on the formation of a constructive partnership between government and the public sector, the private sector, and civil society. TI works in coalitions with actors from all three of these sectors, and it does so at both the national and international level.

Industry Partnerships

Private companies have often been at the forefront of progressive change, leaving the state sector trailing behind. Companies introduced pensions and health care benefits before governments did. Procter & Gamble, for instance, pioneered disability and retirement pensions in 1915. Socially responsible companies build trust with customers, staff, investors, and the community where they work and conduct business.

George W. Merck famously said that "medicine is for the people. It is not for the profits; the profits follow," and Merck and Company, Inc., has taken a lead in distributing some drugs cheaply to poor countries that cannot afford market prices—for instance, Mectizan (ivermectin), a cure for river blindness. However, Merck was one of many companies that were slow to realize the inhumanity of their attempts to protect their patents on drugs against AIDS in South Africa.

A balance must be struck so that patent rights do not jeopardize access to medicines in countries suffering from epidemics. Pharmaceutical companies should also begin to pressure governments to work with them to tackle diseases that affect the poor. Although companies know that they can expect profits more than to pay for their research and investment in cures for rich-country diseases such as arthritis, what are the incentives to tackle tropical diseases?

The incentives include the results—better standards of living and, in turn, prosperous patients with higher life expectancy. But this can happen only if the pharmaceutical industry works together with developed country governments—for example, in waiving patent rights or lowering prices of existing drugs for developing countries.

But companies must engage with recipient governments and civil society in developing countries to ensure that the medicines reach their target—the sick and the needy, not the pockets of corrupt officials—so that there are fewer occasions when vulnerable patients are sold worthless or even dangerous counterfeit drugs.

Public-private partnerships, such as the Global Alliance for TB Drug Development working with Novartis, may be the way forward in shifting the financial risk—and, of course, some of the associated rewards—of product development away from shareholders and onto governments or foundations.

Companies must establish codes of conduct, including detailed rules designed to combat bribery at home or by their subsidiaries abroad. To this end, TI and Social Accountability International have developed, together with companies including BP, Norsk Hydro, Shell, Tata, and General Electric, a set of "Business Principles for Countering Bribery" (http://www.transparency.org/building_coalitions/private_sector/business_principles.html). The proposals include training programs with guidance for all employees to ensure that bribery, direct or indirect, is outlawed.

Working with a multistakeholder international steering committee, the business principles provide for a comprehensive approach to countering bribery by companies, covering both internal policies and practices and external business partners throughout the supply chain.

The pharmaceutical industry needs to join this initiative, to work together with TI and others to honor the dedication of honest professionals saving lives across the globe, and to ensure that the cancer of corruption does not eat away the ethical core values that have made the medical profession the lifesaver we all cherish.

Supporting Civil Society

TI recognizes every year the work of brave individuals who have taken a stand against corruption.

In 2003, one of the winners of the TI Integrity Award was Dora Akunyili, director general of Nigeria's National Agency for Food and Drug Administration and Control (http://www.transparency.org/integrityawards/winners/winners_2003.html#dora). A pharmacologist by training, Akunyili has faced death threats—and at the end of 2003 an assassination attempt—while tackling corrupt practices in the manufacturing, import, and export of drugs, cosmetics, and food products. In particular, she has pursued manufacturers and importers of counterfeit drugs, deemed to be a leading cause of deaths by stroke and heart failure in Nigeria.

In 2002, one of the winners of the TI Integrity Award was Peter S. Schönhöfer, a professor of pharmacology and coeditor of the independent German drugs bulletin, *arznei-telegramm* (http://www.transparency.org/integrityawards/winners/winners.html#schhofer1). Schönhöfer is a resolute critic of corruption in pharmaceutical companies, including practices such as paying honoraria to physicians, interns, and medical department staff to insert nonessential drugs on lists of approved drugs. Schönhöfer has also criticized corrupt medical experts for falsifying scientific data in publications and for not declaring their financial links to pharmaceutical companies. He has warned of the dangers of "pharma-marketing" in corrupting the health care process.

Picking up on the concerns of Schönhöfer, it is critical that hospitals set up appropriate rules, including a written code of conduct, and written policies and procedures on procurement and contracting. (Schönhöfer has also suggested that integrity pacts may be appropriate to safeguard against corruption in the procurement process. For more on integrity pacts, see http://www.transparency.org/integrity_pact/preventing/integ_pacts.html.) Regular ethics training for staff and a complaints hotline with protection for whistleblowers should also be the norm. It is particularly important that any financial contributions by pharmaceutical companies to medical research units be transparent and fully documented, in line with the policies and procedures of the hospital. Sanctions for misdeeds must be sufficient to act as a deterrent.

The insights of Schönhöfer and the bravery of Akunyili offer a challenge to the pharmaceutical companies to join with other stakeholders, including government watchdogs. Pharmaceutical companies need to ensure the integrity of their industry and to save the lives put at threat by the less scrupulous. From TI's point of view, civil society support for greater commitment to transparency can make a tremendous difference in health care outcomes.

Anticorruption Is Pro–Global Health

Protesters within the antiglobalization movement charge that multinational companies behave irresponsibly around the world, exploiting the environment and exploiting cheap labor in developing countries or, as in *The Constant Gardener*, exploiting poor patients as guinea pigs for drug experiments. When pharmaceutical companies make payments to doctors in developing countries for enrolling patients in trials, medical ethics have clearly been compromised. On the one side, international companies are taking advantage of a low-paid doctor; on the other side, the doctor in turn is abusing the trust of vulnerable patients.

The stakes are high, both for the pharmaceutical companies, which continue to constitute one of the most profitable of all sectors, and for people, especially the poor. Is corruption driving the world's ever-growing spending on drugs? Is it denying developing countries access to medicine and medical treatment? The tentative answer is yes, but more analysis is necessary to track the complex practices that lead to unethical, fraudulent, and corrupt dealings in the health sector and to understand the full impact of these crimes.

For TI, one thing is certain: fighting corruption is good for the world's health. TI is eager to build bridges between civil society and the private sector to pressure governments in both the developed and developing worlds to tackle the systemic problems that leave hospitals underfunded. It is necessary to make sure that medicines are not diverted by corrupt elites and that aid money in the health sector reaches its intended destination. And finally, TI expects the pharmaceutical companies that in many ways are the driving force in modern medicine to face up to their responsibility to raise standards and root out the corrupt practices that exacerbate inequality in global health care provision.

Reference

Le Carré, J. *The Constant Gardener*. New York: Simon and Schuster, 2001.

8

Business Approach to HIV/AIDS Crisis in Africa

Spencer T. King

The International Executive Service Corps (IESC) celebrated its fortieth anniversary in 2004. IESC is a nonprofit organization that focuses on enhancing economic growth in developing countries to provide a better quality of life for the citizens of those countries. The core capacity of IESC is the use of private-sector volunteers to deliver technical assistance and other supporting services. From the inception of IESC in 1964, senior U.S. retired executives have completed more than twenty-five thousand technical and managerial assistance projects in more than 120 countries.

As developing nations strive to compete and develop workforces to match a more focused global economy, IESC has also changed to include new capacities. An example is IESC's "Geek Corps" unit, which addresses the dynamic, ever-expanding requirements of its clients for worldwide information technology. Whereas IESC maintains a skills bank of more than ten thousand "traditional" volunteers to service demand from virtually every sector in a developing country economy, it also maintains a "geek" skills bank database of more than sixteen hundred volunteers to address the technology sector. In the former case, the "average" volunteer is retired and fifty-eight years old, and in the latter, the geek volunteer is still employed and thirty years old.

In keeping with our strategy to evolve with the changing dynamics of global economies, IESC has undertaken a new initiative to coordinate business solutions and support activities to deal with the medical and humanitarian crisis of HIV/AIDS (human immunodeficiency virus–acquired immunodeficiency syndrome), especially in sub-Saharan Africa. Recently IESC has developed plans to add a unit of medical volunteers to integrate with its programs worldwide. This blending of American business and medical volunteer capacity will enable IESC to provide a new dimension of services to alleviate the consequences of HIV/AIDS on small enterprises.

IESC Business Support Approach to the HIV/AIDS Crisis

The continuing devastating effect of HIV/AIDS for sub-Saharan Africa defies the imagination, both in scope and complexity. Rightfully so, the donor community's focus has remained on the medical and humanitarian aspects. Treatment, prevention, and community compassion are elements that require enormous funds, energy, and time to deliver. Political and cultural change will be necessary, and in the final analysis, the efficacious distribution of resources will dictate the relative degree of success in the struggle against HIV/AIDS. However, if the allocation of resources is confined to one end of the spectrum—medical treatment and prevention exclusively—what will happen to the productive sector of these developing nations?

For instance, what will the quality of life be for HIV/AIDS victims and their families if no attention is directed toward the totality of the problem? What resources will be available on a sustained basis to allow these individuals to earn a livelihood if the focus is on treatment and prevention to the exclusion of all other factors? Will the constituencies of small and medium enterprises experience a diminished quality of life and reduction of opportunities not just today but in the future? Will this occur because the medical is not coordinated with retraining the private sector to mitigate the enormous impact of HIV/AIDS on businesses? If there is a failure to invest in business planning, legal rights, and HIV/AIDS training and awareness in the workplace, will this not ultimately increase the amount of overall donor assistance necessary to sustain developing nations? If private-sector enterprises cannot cope within the overwhelming context of the HIV/AIDS disaster, what will be left for future generations except an exacerbated dependence on humanitarian aid programs to continually and endlessly meet the challenges not only of HIV/AIDS but also of poverty, non-HIV/AIDS diseases, and a widening gap between these countries and the global economy? These are difficult questions that require a balanced and integrated approach to resolve.

In the final analysis, donor and recipient countries cannot afford to wait while the medical catastrophe is resolved at the expense of quality of life and access to reasonable opportunity for the rest of the population. Solutions must be designed, tested, validated, and modified to match the complexity of the HIV/AIDS pandemic.

Zambia's IESC "Biz/AIDS" Program

Several years ago, IESC vice president for sub-Saharan Africa, Mary Kathryn ("M. K.") Cope, began looking for ways to mitigate the economic effects of HIV/AIDS and other health-related crises on microbusinesses and small and medium-sized businesses. She initiated discussions with the U.S. Agency for International Development (USAID) about developing complementary programmatic approaches to provide a more holistic, complete response to the AIDS pandemic. These discussions led to the establishment of USAID-funded programs called "Biz/AIDS."

Biz/AIDS began in 2004 as an integrated program designed to alleviate the effects of HIV/AIDS on economic development. The program provides targeted training for small businesses in three specific areas:

- Business planning

- Basic awareness training in HIV/AIDS, malaria, and other critical health issues and workplace training on HIV/AIDS

- Legal rights and opportunities

The first tier of the Biz/AIDS program focuses on business planning for small and medium enterprises (SMEs) composed of ten to fifty employees. SMEs constitute a significant part of national employment in sub-Saharan Africa, and companies of this size are particularly vulnerable to a serious business crisis. HIV/AIDS epitomizes individual crises of dramatic proportions that literally wipe out families, individuals, and companies. Often the resources, skills, experience, and commercial competence are not efficiently passed on to viable successors. Therefore, employment opportunities are lost; businesses require reinvestment basically to start all over again; revenue flows that could support better local government initiatives are diminished; and ultimately, the quality of life is lessened for the entire society. Zambian businesses recognized the dilemma of this dynamic and began to articulate requests for technical assistance. The first part of the Biz/AIDS program, business planning, provides Zambian SMEs with the following:

- Business risk assessments

- Strategic business plans to minimize the risk

- Simple business skills training to ultimately implement the strategic business plans

The second tier of the Biz/AIDS program is designed to offer basic information to Zambian SMEs on HIV/AIDS, malaria, and other catastrophic diseases and also training on HIV/AIDS in the workplace. Biz/AIDS proposes better use of existing health programs and resources to enhance prevention, detection, counseling, and treatment. To avoid redundancy, it is essential for Biz/AIDS to carefully analyze the appropriate interventions for specific businesses. The program assures another layer of professional IESC firm-level assistance to continually promote and support practices that allow SMEs to cope with the effects of HIV/AIDS in the workplace.

Although HIV/AIDS has and will create massive human and institutional suffering, there are always better ways to address the problems to lessen the negative effects. The philosophy of IESC Biz/AIDS is that it is important to coordinate with and inform businesses *before* they are significantly affected by the pandemic. Preparation for possible direct exposure to this disease will better protect assets, job security of employees, and the extension of benefits to families and society in general. The Zambian SMEs, particularly in rural areas, are the most vulnerable to the ravages of HIV/AIDS. Simply stated, if they are not aware, prepared, and otherwise empowered with succession plans, cross-training modules, and protection of acquired assets, they can be devastated. Economic opportunities will never be fully realized because outside buyers, potential partners, and possible foreign direct investment are dissuaded from investing because of perceived risk.

The third area that the Biz/AIDS program addresses is providing access to existing legal programs and resources to ensure that SMEs understand all of the legal requirements for businesses in crisis. Biz/AIDS facilitates wills and business succession plans, insurance programs, health care schemes, human resource development, and other mechanisms to sustain SMEs through serious challenges to their existence.

Biz/AIDS Development Process

This three-part Biz/AIDS program did not emanate from a concept alone but rather from long-term IESC experience in sub-Saharan Africa. The Biz/AIDS proposal illustrates the ability of IESC to provide solutions for private-sector economic growth. The original IESC Cooperative Agreement with USAID began in 1992, with a primary focus on supporting the privatization process being deployed by the Zambian government in the early 1990s. Subsequently, the "Livingstone Linkages" program was developed as a result of the changing economic climate in Zambia and USAID's shifting strategic objectives.

Since the start of the Livingstone Linkages program in February 2001, IESC has worked with more than three hundred SMEs in Zambia to help them grow through "horizontal" linkages as well as the more common development approach of "vertical" linkages. Review of growth opportunities in the country has identified tourism as the fastest-growing industry in Zambia, with Livingstone as one of the most promising destinations. Each business in the travel and tourism industry affects at least nine other businesses, including printing and publishing, utilities, financial services, furnishings, security services, transportation, promotion, computers, laundry services, and so on. To improve the tourism industry, all other businesses that feed into it would need to be improved simultaneously. Therefore, IESC linked small businesses vertically into the tourism industry and also provided valuable technical assistance through IESC volunteers to ancillary (horizontal) businesses. (Incidentally, the IESC volunteer-donated services in effect double the "bang for the buck." Volunteers work on a cost basis, forgoing the consulting fee. Their contribution dramatically extends the foreign and technical assistance dollar.)

The Livingstone Linkages program ended in 2002, with the program lessons providing the foundation for IESC's follow-on "Copperlink Program," designed and implemented for small businesses in the Zambian Copperbelt. IESC's strategic partner in this program was the District Business Association in Livingstone. IESC conducted numerous workshops throughout the Copperlink Program with an additional component, "HIV/AIDS in the Workplace."

In this collaborative process, small business experts in Zambia used IESC's SME *Business Survival Planning Workbook* (2004) to walk business owners through a process of identifying their business assets, ensuring support for business management during absences, cross-training employees, and creating support networks in times of crisis and transition. Templates for legal rights and opportunities training were developed and delivered to participants.

Although IESC had incorporated elements of the Biz/AIDS program into the Copperlink Program, it became impossible to ignore that the businesses we were working with were being profoundly affected by HIV/AIDS. Although there were programs in Zambia providing HIV/AIDS-in-the-workplace training from the health perspective, these programs had been working only with the largest companies in the country (one thousand–plus employees) and had not addressed the economic effects of the disease. Microenterprises and SMEs were completely left out of this process.

The ultimate point of the Biz/AIDS initiative as a separate, stand-alone program is that HIV/AIDS has become more than a health issue: it has become a development issue. "Our efforts began with one volunteer project," said M. K. Cope. "IESC Volunteer Expert Joan Sherman looked at the impact of HIV/AIDS on the businesses in Livingstone and worked with a U.N. volunteer to help businesses develop a strategy to withstand the economic impact of the disease. Joan and several volunteers started to provide training in employee cross-training, and established someone to be in charge of each business in case the owner became incapacitated. (In many cases, this was the wife of the business owner)," according to Cope. "Finally, where able, the volunteers helped the business owners to establish a will to prevent the business assets from being stripped if the owner died" (personal communication, phone, May 2004).

From this early work, IESC developed a training program and tool kit. Since 2001, IESC has worked directly with approximately 180 companies to implement the Biz/AIDS methodology. These companies come from eleven communities in the rural and periurban areas of Zambia, including Livingstone, Petauke, Zambezi, and eight communities in the Copperbelt region. IESC has also worked with eleven District Business Associations to train them in the Biz/AIDS method and to implement the method in their businesses. To date, we estimate that the training has directly affected three hundred individuals.

On May 13, 2004, USAID awarded a stand-alone program to IESC to formally apply the Biz/AIDS method in Zambia. The Biz/AIDS program manager will be based in the capital, Lusaka, and regional hubs will be established in Choma (Southern Province), Mongu (Western Province), and Chipata (Eastern Province on the border with Malawi). The Zambia Chamber of Small and Medium Business Associations and its member District Business Associations will continue to be our partners in this program.

IESC also has a proposal under submission to USAID South Africa for a yearlong program to implement Biz/AIDS with the South Africa Business Coalition on HIV/AIDS (SABCOHA), a member of the Global Business Coalition on HIV/AIDS. SABCOHA has already developed a tool kit and method for businesses with fifty to two hundred employees. The Biz/AIDS South Africa program will be working with three to five small business associations and their members with one to forty-nine employees in a Johannesburg area township, most likely Alexadra or Soweto. The businesses with one to nineteen employees will be trained using the IESC method developed in Zambia. A separate method and tool kit will be developed for businesses with twenty to forty-nine employees during the twelve-month pilot program.

We anticipate that the national and regional implications of the Zambia and South Africa Biz/AIDS programs will be evident in the short term. Helping SMEs to prepare for and cope with the effects of HIV/AIDS on their businesses does not diminish the needs and priorities of the health treatment issue itself. Rather, IESC offers complementary and comprehensive support mechanisms to small businesses to deal with the crisis. Much more should be considered to force "thinking out of the box" and provide innovative solutions for the HIV/AIDS pandemic crisis.

IESC continually seeks to leverage its resources and those of USAID entrusted to IESC. Public-private partnerships can provide great advantages, using multinational drug companies to contribute to USAID funding mechanisms like global development alliances. Business coalitions such as SABCOHA are natural partners to develop strategies that have an effect on business development.

As mentioned earlier, IESC itself, now beginning its forty-first year of existence, is expanding resources to better resolve emerging needs of developing countries. Discussions are under way to combine our firm-level, person-to-person capability with volunteer physicians in preventive medicine for new, on-site programs in training and awareness. The IESC business approach augments and leverages the efforts and funding flowing through the health pipeline—and also the development pipeline—to deliver innovative services to empower SMEs in the fight against HIV/AIDS. Moreover, the IESC solution delivers the additional benefit of donated volunteer services that extend scarce foreign aid dollars. That is IESC's organizational contribution to a crisis of epic proportions.

We hope to mitigate the devastating effects in sub-Saharan Africa from HIV/AIDS in a societal, holistic manner. We recognize that IESC plays only a small role in the great challenge of fighting HIV/AIDS, but ultimately, our modest contributions will save precious resources, lessen human suffering, and provide for greater civil stability internationally.

Reference

International Executive Service Corps. *SME Business Survival Planning Workbook*. Proprietary IESC Internal Program Document, Washington, D.C.: International Executive Service Corps, 2004.

9

. . . .

Health in the Developing World
Achieving the Millennium Development Goals

Jeffrey D. Sachs

A revolution in public health thinking and practice is under way as part of a broader campaign to end extreme poverty. There is a growing recognition worldwide that the time has come to fulfill the long-standing pledge to make health services available for all, including the poorest of the poor. Poor countries around the world are taking bold steps to scale up the health services in their countries. They are now looking to the rich countries to hold up their end of the bargain.

The Millennium Development Goals (MDGs), the international objectives on poverty reduction adopted by the world community in 2000, provide the broad context for this revolution in thinking and practice. The MDGs place a central focus on public health, in recognition of the fact that improvements in public health are vital not only in their own right but also to break the poverty trap of the world's poorest economies. A significant number of the MDGs are explicitly about health: reducing child mortality by two-thirds by 2015; reducing maternal mortality by three-quarters by 2015; controlling the great pandemic diseases of AIDS (acquired

This article is adapted from an address to the Second Global Consultation of the Commission on Macroeconomics and Health in Geneva, October 29, 2003.

It is reprinted with permission of *The Bulletin of the World Health Organization*, Dec. 2004, 82(12).

immunodeficiency syndrome), malaria, and tuberculosis; giving access to safe drinking water and sanitation; and alleviating hunger and undernutrition. Moreover, the first MDG, to reduce by half the proportion of the population in extreme poverty ("dollar-a-day" poverty) by 2015, cannot conceivably be accomplished if the health goals are not achieved. Societies burdened by a large number of sick and dying individuals cannot escape from poverty.

The MDGs emerged from the Millennium Declaration adopted by all countries of the United Nations. They provide political leverage for health ministries to use within their own societies and in negotiations with the donor world. Not only did the world subscribe to these goals but also the United Nations (U.N.) member governments reaffirmed these commitments several times since, including at the International Conference on Financing for Development (Monterrey, Mexico, March 2002) and the World Summit on Sustainable Development (Johannesburg, South Africa, September 2002). In the Monterrey Consensus, the rich and poor countries adopted a compact. The poor countries accepted the responsibilities of good governance, serious policy design, transparency, and openness to real implementation, and the rich countries accepted the responsibilities of greatly increased donor financing. Specifically, paragraph 42 of the Monterrey Consensus reads: "We urge developed countries that have not done so to make concrete efforts towards the target of 0.7 percent of gross national product (GNP) as official development assistance to developing countries." Honoring that commitment would signify an increase in donor aid from roughly U.S.\$70 billion per year to U.S.\$210 billion per year, in view of today's donor GNP of some U.S.\$30 trillion at current prices and exchange rates.

Keeping in mind that the rich countries as well as the poor signed the Monterrey Consensus, the amount of additional funding needed to solve the global health crisis should be readily available. Developing countries should not be reticent about making clear that they need more financial help, without which they will be a danger to themselves and to richer countries. If malaria and AIDS are not brought under control, if children are dying of respiratory tract infections because they breathe wood smoke inside huts for lack of modern cooking fuels, if they are not drinking safe water, the result is a tragedy not only for the poor world but also a danger for the rich world. The rich countries have to understand that there is no chance for political and social stability in the world if they do not help the poor to fight the war against disease. Disease leads to extreme poverty; extreme poverty leads to political instability; political instability leads to state failure; and state failure, alas, leads to violence, criminality, and havens for terrorism, not to mention the international transmission of disease itself.

The Commission on Macroeconomics and Health (CMH) found that roughly U.S.$27 billion per year (at 2001 prices and exchange rates) would be needed from donors as of 2007 to enable the poorest countries to deliver basic lifesaving health services. At today's prices and exchange rates, that is probably closer to U.S.$30 billion per year. The figure represents around 0.1 percent of donor income, that is, ten cents per every hundred dollars of rich-world income. Because the current level of official development assistance is 0.25 percent and the promised level is 0.7 percent, the gap—equal to around 0.45 percent of donor GNP—would easily accommodate the increased spending in health services.

The common objection to plans for increased aid to scale up health systems is "absorptive capacity," that is, the human, infrastructure, and macroeconomic constraints that may limit a country's ability to effectively absorb aid. In considering this issue, however, the CMH and now the U.N. Millennium Project, an advisory project to U.N. Secretary-General Kofi Annan that I have the honor to direct, have concluded that developing countries can absorb substantial increases of assistance if directed toward investments in health, especially if those investments are phased in over time in a sensible manner and according to an overall plan. In terms of macroeconomics, increased health investments financed by donor assistance will not destabilize countries but will actually give a tremendous boost to productivity and to their ability to achieve economic growth. The main issues are not macroeconomic but rather sectoral: ensuring that increased spending on health actually leads to increases in the capacity of the health system to deliver health services. This can be accomplished with well-designed plans for scaling up health services that extend over several years.

For poor countries to obtain more donor financing for health, they should take four steps. First, they must have an overall strategy for scaling up health services. Many ministries of health have already developed strategies for increasing the coverage of health services but have often been told by donors to shelve the plans because they are too expensive. Now it is time to take those strategies off the shelf, if they exist, or to make new plans if the first step has not yet been taken. The strategies should be ambitious enough to meet the health MDGs and to offer essential health services to the whole society, with special attention to the needs of the poorest of the poor. The rich countries must understand that the time to duck behind the excuse that the plan is "too expensive" is long past, given the commitments that those countries have made repeatedly in recent years.

Second, detailed plans of implementation are needed, especially a sequence of investments in physical capital (clinics, hospitals, training centers) and in health professionals. The implementation plans must be logistically thorough, focusing on details in each major area of public health: how communities will be reached when there are not enough doctors, what kind of community health workers must be trained, what logistics systems will be in place for managing the supply of medicines, and so forth. The plans should present with great care the kinds of human resource development—physicians, nurses, community health workers, health sector managers—that will be required and when.

Third, there has to be a financing plan that combines additional resources from donors and from domestic tax revenues. The CMH agreed that all developing countries should be allocating more of the national budgetary revenues to health. Specifically, as an overall guideline, the CMH called for an increase of one percentage point of GNP in annual health spending in public-sector budgets by 2007 and an increase of two percentage points of GNP in annual health spending by 2015. For middle-income countries, such an increase in budget spending on health might be enough to ensure universal access to basic health services. For the poorest countries, however, added donor assistance will be vital.

Consider the case of an impoverished sub-Saharan African country with a GNP of $300 per person per year as of 2003. The cost of universal access to basic health services might be around $36 per person per year, or roughly 12 percent of GNP. Currently, budgetary spending might be on the order of only $3 per person per year, or 1 percent of GNP. According to CMH guidelines, the domestic effort should rise by one percentage point of GNP as of 2007 and two percentage points of GNP as of 2015. Suppose that per capita income is rising at 2 percent per year. In 2007, GNP per capita is around $325. Public spending on health should by then be 2 percent of GNP, according to the CMH guidelines, or $6.50 per year, leaving a shortfall of $29.50 that would have to be made up by donors. By 2015, GNP per capita would be around $380, and public spending on health would be 3 percent of GNP, or $11.40, leaving a shortfall relative to $36 per capita of $24.60, again requiring donor assistance to fill the financing gap. Can the rich world really begrudge the poor this amount of help? The United States currently spends about U.S.$5,000 per person to run its health system: health systems need computers, information systems, management, physicians, and nurses. Donor agencies should not expect developing countries to run a health system for U.S.$5 per capita and then accuse them of being inefficient when the system does not work. Salaries have to be good enough to keep qualified health personnel in the health posts rather than migrating in search of better prospects. Poor countries cannot afford a good system without help from the richer ones. The fact is that the donors would hardly notice it—a few billion dollars a year is a rounding error in the U.S. budget; yet, millions of people could be saved with that money.

The financing plans that developing countries will present at consultative discussions, or to the International Monetary Fund and the World Bank, should explain that funding essential health services requires not the few million dollars that they have been receiving for the health sector but hundreds of millions or perhaps $1 billion for large countries. It should remind donors that they have promised on many occasions to provide the needed funding.

The fourth step is advocacy. Developing countries' plans must be transparently designed, and they have to involve not only health ministries but also civil society: mission hospitals, nongovernmental organizations, community centers, and the country coordinating mechanisms that bring together all these critical stakeholders.

These plans must be brought into the real donor processes. Developing countries prepare Poverty Reduction Strategy Papers (PRSPs) for submission to the International Monetary Fund and the World Bank. Health ministers must start getting bold health sector programs into these PRSPs, based on real financing needs. Above all, the programs have to be ambitious enough to achieve the MDGs because those are what the world signed up to and what (at the minimum) the PRSPs aim to accomplish. Countries have to plan to get on track to reduce mortality for children aged five years and younger by two-thirds by 2015. If getting on track means tripling the development assistance needed for health, they must say so.

In addition to the PRSPs, another important donor process revolves around the Global Fund to Fight AIDS, Tuberculosis and Malaria. Most developing countries have programs that are too small. Countries have to resist the pressure from donors who are trying to get programs scaled down and instead present ambitious, realistic plans on a national scale to the Global Fund: not what the donors say can be paid for but what is really needed.

This is an important time. Poor countries are increasingly clamoring for results and have plans to achieve them. This is a moment of truth. Do we live in a civilized world with a truly global community? Do we acknowledge our common humanity and understand that it is uncivilized to let people die for the lack of a small sum that could easily be mobilized? Do we understand the dangers to the entire world if we fail to act?

References

Report of the Commission on Macroeconomics and Health. Geneva: World Health Organization, 2001.

Report of the International Conference for Development, 2002. Monterrey, Mexico, March 2002. New York: United Nations. Available: http://www.un.org/esa/ffd/aconf198–11.pdf. Accessed: Jan. 10, 2005.

Part III

Creating Networks and Partnerships
and Planning Change from Within

10

Leadership and Management
for Improving Global Health

Frances Hesselbein

Today we share a dream that lies before us: healthy children everywhere, healthy families, healthy communities—a healthy global society where equal access to health care is the norm, not the exception.

Still, it is only a vision, a dream. Community health care professionals and the leaders of health care agencies, groups, hospitals, universities, and organizations are called to mobilize around a powerful vision of the future: equal access to primary health care for all of our people, in our own country and in countries all over the world. The goal of healthy children everywhere remains a dream until leaders at every level of every organization, agency, hospital, and university working to improve global health care to serve all of our people mobilize.

We are fellow travelers on a long journey toward an uncertain future where the challenges will be exceeded only by the opportunities to lead, to innovate, to advocate, to change lives, and to shape and redefine the future. Wide disparities, limited resources, and tenuous times form the context of our response, the background for this essential battle. The journey calls for spirited, inspired leaders of change. As we move into a tenuous future, our mission, the star we steer by, will be our greatest protector; the values we live by, our greatest security; and innovation—the indispensable, common imperative for leaders of change—will chart the way in a world forever changed, a world at war.

In a seminal article in the November 3–9, 2001, issue of *The Economist*, Peter Drucker's wisdom spreads across twenty incredible pages. One observation he makes is most relevant to our global health challenge: seeing the organization as a change agent. We are used to hearing that you and I must be change agents. But as Drucker writes, "To survive and succeed, every organization will have to turn itself into a change agent. The most effective way to manage change successfully is to create it. But experience has shown that grafting innovation onto a traditional enterprise does not work. The enterprise has to become a change agent. Instead of seeing change as a threat, its people will come to consider it as an opportunity" (2001, p. 19). Drucker delivers a powerful leadership imperative: making our global health organizations "change agents." This challenges us to exercise tough discipline in moving innovation across the enterprise and getting our house in order as we hurtle into a tenuous future. In this crucible of massive societal change, there is no time to negotiate with nostalgia.

As leaders, we know that some of the practices of the past are not relevant to the present we are living and the future we envision. Nowhere is change as rapid as in the field of health care. So leaders of change will find the courage to throw out the old hierarchy, along with outmoded, irrelevant policies, practices, procedures, and assumptions that limit our ability to bring essential health care to all children, all families, all communities, and all countries.

We ban that old structure chart with people in boxes. We purge the vocabulary of up and down, top and bottom; we learn to move across the organization and understand the wisdom of teams. We practice a flexible, fluid, circular management. We are "managing in a world that is round" (Hesselbein, 1996).

When we move people out of the old boxes and match our language with the new structure, we liberate the human spirit. We look around us: human needs and health needs are escalating; traditional resources are diminishing. Then we challenge the gospel of what is. We have the courage to challenge every policy, practice, and assumption; we challenge the status quo. This is tough to do but essential if we are to get our house in order, to be relevant in a turbulent future.

One of the most difficult tasks is "planned abandonment"— Drucker's term—abandonment of what worked yesterday may work today but has little relevance for the future. We ask, will this policy, project, practice, or initiative be viable in 2010? If not, we practice planned abandonment. We put our house in order because we are determined to provide health care for all of the world's people.

So, with a sense of urgency, we challenge the status quo because we live in a world where many governments at many levels are abandoning the health and human services they once delivered or supported. Business alone is unable to provide these essential services governments are relinquishing.

The nongovernmental organization (NGO) and nonprofit sectors are facing new and enormous expectations that somehow this third sector—this social sector—alone will be able to provide the essential health services to children, families, and communities that the other two sectors are unable to deliver.

The day of the partnership is upon us. And if we share a vision—and our vision of the future is a country, a world of healthy children everywhere, healthy families, good schools, decent housing, work that dignifies, all embraced by the healthy, diverse, inclusive community—then leaders of change, leaders of the future must move beyond the walls. They must find partners, alliances, and collaborations and build the healthy, cohesive community as energetically as they built the bureau, the hospital, the organization, the agency, and the enterprise within the walls.

For the first time, all three sectors are beginning to acknowledge that alone they cannot meet the burgeoning health needs of the global society. In these new partnerships, a new passion for eliminating disparities could lead the way. The power of mission, the power of example, the power of inclusion, the power of collaboration can move us from where we are to where we are determined to be. We know we cannot sit at our desks and say, "Let there be global health care" and have anything happen. It happens when all of us together all over the world mobilize around a common mission of bringing health care to our global family.

I cannot forget that in this world every night millions of children go to bed hungry. This is intolerable. We know that a child who is hungry has difficulty learning and growing, and ten or fifteen years from now a society will pay a price far greater than feeding those children now when we deal with the problems of a whole cohort of young people with inadequate nutrition, poor schooling, and lack of primary health care.

One of the signs of hope for a brighter future is a new kind of collaboration as leaders in all three sectors are coming together, called to mobilize around critical issues. Everything leaders in this field are doing converges into a new leadership imperative: every word, every act, and every initiative tested against the imperative of healing, changing lives, and building the healthy community. Part of that new leadership imperative is global, with powerful advocacy for change in a world that has changed forever. It begins with a vision.

With new alliances and partnerships in collaboration, we can transform the world. In these new partnerships, there is new hope. Leaders must lead from the front and lead beyond the walls into the future. The challenge: How do we mobilize our partners in all three sectors to respond to our vision of the future? All of us are struggling with the seismic transformation of the global society. In our own way and in our own organization, each of us takes our own small part of the global challenge of basic heath care for all.

We are called to see change, never as a threat, but always as a remarkable opportunity to reach a new level of relevance, a new level of significance. This is a call for leadership beyond skills or skills set. It requires the art of principled leadership.

Our times call for leaders of quality and character who have a moral compass that works full-time, leaders who are healers and unifiers and who keep the faith.

Leaders in all three sectors are finding that the old answers do not fit the new questions. Across the three sectors, it is common questions, common challenges, and a call for principled leadership. It is all about leadership.

The dream that lies before us—equal access to primary health care for every child and every man and woman around the world—is only a dream until leaders respond to a common vision. We are just beginning the long journey toward equal access to global health. The health care challenges that lie ahead will be exceeded only by remarkable opportunities to change lives and build healthy communities with equal access to health care around the world. It all begins with leadership, leaders at every level of every enterprise in every sector—business, government, and the NGO-voluntary-nonprofit sectors—mobilizing around a common mission. It will call leaders, wherever they are, to take their share of this global challenge and work together to find common ground with common goals and common language. Improving global health is the critical challenge to leaders in all three sectors around the world.

Today we are called to redefine leadership, just as we must redefine the organization. Leaders learn leadership definitions from others even as we work to define leadership on our own terms. We define the art of leadership in our own lives as we embody our values and principles in our behavior and our performance and as we define and practice leadership in the future.

In the end, we must find the language that expresses our own leadership beliefs because language is the enduring gift of the leader. My personal definition of leadership when I was with Girl Scouts of the United States of America and today is: "Leadership is a matter of how to be, not how to do!" We spend most of our lives learning how to do and teaching others how to do; yet, in the end it is the quality and character of the leader that determine the performance and the results.

The future is in our hands. If we do not invest today in the health care of all of our children, the other investments we make will be irrelevant. The dream that lies before us begins with healthy children everywhere, and it is only a dream until leaders in all three sectors respond to this call. It is a call to leaders of quality and character to put our houses in order, to mobilize around the mission—equal access to quality health care for all—to move beyond the walls and in collaboration, leading from the dream we share to the healthy future our world deserves.

References

Drucker, P. "The Next Society: A Survey of the Near Future." *Economist*, Nov. 3–9, 2001, *361*(8246), 3–20.

Hesselbein, F. "Managing in a World That Is Round." *Leader to Leader*, Fall 1996, *2*, 6–8.

11

Creating Public Health Alliances

The American Cancer Society Experience

John R. Seffrin

When the third cholera epidemic of the century struck London in 1849, medical officials were at a loss. At the crest of the epidemic, the neighborhood at the intersection of Broad and Cambridge streets was especially hard hit. More than five hundred people fell ill with the disease in a ten-day period, and John Snow, a physician, set out to discover why. He spoke with the victims about their daily habits, and one clear commonality emerged: the overwhelming majority drew their water from the public well on Broad Street. Snow convinced authorities that the well was the likely source of the outbreak, and they rendered it inoperable by removing the pump handle. The number of new cholera cases dropped dramatically, and the epidemic in the area abated (DeSalle, 1999).

Snow's campaign is the first reported occurrence of a public health crisis being curtailed by a simple action based on scientific inquiry. Unfortunately, the public health crises of the twenty-first century are so complex that we can no longer rely on "pump-handle" solutions. Instead, the complicated medical, social, political, and economic issues surrounding modern public health demand that governments, organizations, and individuals work together in a concerted effort to identify and execute effective solutions.

Review of the Literature

The major public health concerns of our time are as much matters of public policy as they are of research and discovery. This parallel to advocacy efforts offers many lessons to public health collaborations. In public health as in advocacy, critical mass counts. Advocacy coalitions unite disparate voices into a single clear signal that lawmakers can easily understand. Public health collaborations bring together a variety of objectives, agendas, and methods into one organized, effective effort.

In "Building and Maintaining Advocacy Coalitions," a chapter in the *Democracy Owners Manual* (2001), Schultz identifies benefits that are equally applicable to public health collaborations:

- Partnerships that unite organizations with diverse images and support bases represent a cross-section of the population that is influential with policymakers, the media, and other leaders who are critical to the accomplishment of the groups' goals.

- No one organization holds all the necessary resources or all the brilliant ideas. Partnerships allow the groups to pool their resources and develop a more complete tool kit, and they arrive at the freshest, most innovative ideas through discussion and debate with like-minded colleagues.

- Partners can divide responsibilities and match them to each organization's strengths so there is less duplication of effort.

- Partnerships unite local, state, and national efforts; local organizations gain increased influence beyond their own communities, and state and national organizations gain increased grassroots support.

- Partnerships allow veteran and novice movement leaders to learn from each other. New leaders learn from the veterans' experience, and seasoned leaders are exposed to fresh perspectives, ideas, and enthusiasm.

- Creating change is a slow—and often frustrating—process, but partnerships generate a sense of purpose and commitment that keeps motivation high.

A 1998 study in conjunction with the World Health Organization (WHO) confirms these and other benefits of collaboration for health promotion (Gillies, 1998). A review of best practices from six WHO regions showed that public health alliances provide the communication network necessary to build social capital. Defined as trust in society generated by civic and social engagement, social capital is a proven determinant of health and well-being. When such alliances cross lay and professional boundaries to unite public, private, and nongovernmental organizations in a common effort, sustainable improvements in public health result.

Collaborations that effectively share power, authority, responsibility, and accountability are successful in promoting health-related behavior change. They can also positively affect public policies that correct health inequalities based on poverty, unemployment, and homelessness. The participating regions' best practices clearly indicate that collaboration among public health organizations positively affects the health, and also the civic and social well-being, of individuals, families, and communities.

Making Collaboration an Organizational Priority

We at the American Cancer Society embrace collaboration as critical to our mission's success, but the enormous return on investment of public health alliances was not always so patently obvious. After the

National Cancer Act of 1971 was passed, few organizations beyond the American Cancer Society and the National Cancer Institute were devoted exclusively to fighting the disease. As other cancer control organizations formed and as the country's understanding of cancer grew, it became clear that there would be no single solution. Long-term research into cancer prevention, treatment, and patient support would be necessary, and it was obvious that no one organization could control the disease on its own. If we were to make timely progress against cancer, we would have to be united in the effort.

We recognized that if services were to be improved, information gaps filled, and unnecessary duplication of effort eliminated, we would have to cooperate with others in productive ways. Working with others certainly has inherent challenges, but the cost of not doing so is far too great.

We set about making collaboration an organizational priority, and in 1998, the American Cancer Society adopted the following as an official guiding principle: "Efforts should be increased at all levels of the American Cancer Society for working with other organizations and agencies to achieve our common cancer control goals and objectives." We assigned full-time staff specifically to manage our collaboration efforts, and we began to develop a set of criteria to guide them. The society follows these quality standards for collaboration:

- Determine that the goal of the collaboration is linked to the society's goals and priorities.

- Determine that the goal can most effectively be achieved through working together, rather than by any one organization working alone.

- Fully understand potential collaborators' mission, goals, structure, values, policies, limitations, expectations, constituencies, organizational culture, and previous collaboration with the society.

- Consider how the collaboration will affect other collaborations or other agendas and goals of the society, both in the short term and over the long term.

- Determine that the society's role in the collaboration is an appropriate role given our resources and priorities.

- Know the level and depth of the commitment required for the collaboration.

- Determine that the collaboration adheres to the established values of the society.

- Seek to facilitate rather than control the collaborative process.

- Mutually develop a clearly defined vision, mission, goals, roles, responsibilities, and operating procedures that are agreed on by all participants and put in writing.

- Disclose to the group any issue on which we cannot compromise.

- Fully share in the risks, responsibilities, and rewards of the effort.

- Obtain the full endorsement of the appropriate society leadership.

- Apply other society quality standards as appropriate.

- Provide a volunteer, staff person, or both as the society's representative who has adequate skills and experience, the appropriate support and resources, and a clear understanding of the ability to make commitments on the organization's behalf.

- Regularly review the collaboration's progress and function to determine whether or not the society should continue to participate.

Since making collaboration an organizational priority, the American Cancer Society has become involved in scores of partnerships that are daily increasing our effectiveness and that are helping us make significant strides toward achieving our mission. We partner with the National Cancer Institute on more than three dozen collaborations focused on cancer research, education, prevention, early detection, and patient services and on tobacco cessation and eliminating health care disparities. In partnership with the Centers for Disease Control and Prevention, the society participates in another four dozen projects focused on other aspects of these same core areas.

Other partnerships are smaller in scale but no less influential. We are working with the Health Resources and Services Administration to increase cancer screening for the medically underserved. We work with U.S. Department of Agriculture's extension agents to deliver cancer prevention and early detection messages to traditionally hard-to-reach populations. We help the American College of Surgeons keep physicians up to date on the most current screening guidelines, and we work with the National Comprehensive Cancer Network to produce current cancer prevention and treatment guidelines in lay terms. Pharmacia partners with us on a National Colorectal Cancer Roundtable. And thousands of employers nationwide collaborate with us to spread the word about cancer prevention and early detection to their employees.

These and other efforts have turned the American Cancer Society into a far more strategic and constructive organization, one that is an equal partner with the government and for-profit sectors in the quest to eradicate cancer. One example of such an effort that is reaping significant public health dividends for the cancer community is C=Change, the National Dialogue on Cancer, formed in 1998, as C=Change connects key leaders in the fight against cancer from the public, private, and nonprofit sectors to work together to eliminate the disease as a major health problem at the earliest possible time.

Analysis of Two Successful Collaborative Efforts

In 1996, the American Cancer Society's board of directors established ambitious goals for 2015: to reduce cancer mortality by 50 percent and cancer incidence by 25 percent. We quickly realized that we could achieve these goals on schedule only by collaborating with others. We identified a group of potential partners whose strategic plans embraced similar goals, and we established a coalition with a clear set of goals. The driving tactic behind C=Change is to unite more than 150 diverse groups from every sector around a common goal and to work together to move forward in achieving it.

The C=Change's goals are necessarily ambitious: its long-term goal is to eradicate cancer as a major public health problem at the earliest possible time, and its one-year goal is to prevent an additional one million new cancer cases and an additional five hundred thousand cancer deaths. The partners committed to seven principles necessary to achieve such lofty goals:

- To promote research as the engine that drives our understanding of cancer

- To close the gap between knowledge learned through research and application of that knowledge in the community to benefit all people

- To help collaborating partners work together on issues that cannot be addressed as effectively alone

- To reach all people—especially those at greatest cancer risk—including minorities and the medically underserved

- To promote cancer prevention and early detection and to provide access to quality health care that will enhance cancer patients' quality of life

- To reenergize the national fight against cancer

- To work to end tobacco use among both youth and adults

We recognized that it would be necessary to develop a strong and diverse group of partners if we were to effect such sweeping change, so we established membership criteria for the coalition. Potential partners must have the capacity to significantly contribute to achieving the C=Change's mission. They must be willing and able to provide direct or in-kind support to the coalition and to demonstrate personal and organizational commitment to its goals. Each prospective partner organization must come from a category or discipline necessary to ensure the desired balance of representatives from the public, private, and nonprofit sectors. Each must be recommended by three peers in the field, and each must commit to be an advocate for the group and its mission.

To ensure that each of these members receives equal partnership status and unfettered participation opportunities, C=Change has a formal funding, meeting, and communication structure. Although the American Cancer Society provided the initial funding for the collaboration, as the group grew, the partners collectively established a resource acquisition campaign to obtain external funding. By registering as a 501(c)3 organization, each member can join in the effort to raise the funds necessary to achieve the mission. The full group meets for semiannual collaborating-partner meetings. To enhance effectiveness and foster relationships and communication, the C=Change also offers partners the opportunity to participate in the work groups of their choice. These smaller teams meet throughout the year and report progress, issues for resolution, and proposed strategies to the full group at the semiannual meetings. The full group will discuss each work group's report and build consensus on next steps.

Each of the member organizations is reaping the benefits of a successful collaborative effort. Each member possesses strengths from which the other members can learn and grow. Each member learns what the other members are doing to fight cancer, allowing the organization to take leadership in accomplishing goals that are not being addressed so that there is minimal duplication of effort. And each is building relationships throughout the cancer community in all sectors that may not otherwise have been possible.

For the first time in public health history, the C=Change brings together the public, private, and nonprofit sectors in a national forum that allows major cancer leaders to discuss both concerns and opportunities. These groups work together to build consensus about how to wage the war against cancer and how to repair the fragmentation of the cancer community. The group unites organizations in an effort to overcome barriers to progress against cancer, and both the member organizations themselves and the state of public health gain from the relationship.

In addition to the society's wealth of public health partnerships, we have extended our organizational commitment to collaboration to include our substantial advocacy efforts. One Voice Against Cancer (OVAC), formed in 1999, unites more than fifty cancer organizations in a common advocacy initiative that is making momentous strides in the drive to establish cancer as a priority with U.S. lawmakers.

Before 1999, the society's national government relations department had seen firsthand how groups with common interests lost opportunities to fund vital cancer research and application programs by approaching lawmakers with scores of similar—but disjointed— "asks." Although many members of Congress wanted to help, they were often faced with too many choices, and as a result, many important cancer programs were receiving inadequate funding. Recognizing that our basic goal, eradicating cancer, is the same, these fifty competitors cast aside their differences and collaborated to leverage their power collectively and make a greater difference than any one of the organizations could have made on its own.

OVAC delivers a unified message to Congress and the White House about the critical need for increased appropriations to support cancer research and programs. The fifty member groups leverage their individual grassroots advocacy power to convince policymakers to increase funding for the National Institutes of Health, the National Cancer Institute, the National Center on Minority Health and Health Disparities, and the Centers for Disease Control and Prevention. All fifty partners are bound to honor this goal and to work to achieve it however possible. Member groups must follow only one requirement: they must agree to work together toward their shared goal and not to perform any activity that will contravene the group's priorities.

Any cancer or public health group that is willing to commit to OVAC's goal is welcome to join the coalition. There are no other membership requirements, and outreach occurs continually so that all potentially interested organizations with a common agenda know about the opportunity. An independent consultant provides staff support to the coalition, and members are invited to be equal partners in setting the group's priorities and agenda. Groups support the coalition based on their individual financial resources, but each is equally influential in its governance.

Although all members share a common goal, they have differing opinions about how to achieve it, and OVAC has served as a catalyst for spirited debate. Each of the more than fifty partners learns from the perspectives of the others, and all decisions are based on consensus. If the partners cannot agree on an issue, the group does not pursue it.

This level of cooperation is achieved through continual open communication. Each partner participates in an annual meeting to set the coalition's agenda for the coming year. The group determines how to achieve the agenda through frequent conference calls and meetings throughout the year. These meetings are task-oriented and focus on action items the members can carry out together to make progress toward their common objectives.

The partnership has been equally beneficial for both small partners and large ones. All groups benefit from the opportunity to network and share best practices. Larger groups work side by side with smaller groups and learn from them; they might never have had the opportunity to meet otherwise. Smaller groups gain a more visible platform to conduct their efforts and secure positive results on their priority issues.

Whereas OVAC has enriched all its member organizations, its ultimate measure of success is the effect it is having on the fight against cancer. Since 1999, OVAC has helped increase the National Cancer Institute's budget by more than $1 billion, providing crucial funds for the cancer screening, education, treatment, research, and services that are making tangible and lasting progress against the disease. OVAC's united front enhances each organization's ability to attain the funding necessary to triumph over cancer.

Through these and other successful collaborations, the American Cancer Society has learned that group effort is the most effective way to achieve maximum delivery of our mission. As our collaborative efforts have evolved over time, we have learned lessons that continue to shape and strengthen our current and future partnerships.

Lessons Learned

The first step toward establishing an effective collaboration is to set a goal and identify partners who can help you successfully realize it. It is not necessary that the partners you identify share your mission; it is only necessary that they share your interest in achieving the specific goal at hand. It is often productive to collaborate with groups with which you may otherwise have little in common. Taking risks that may be counterintuitive in collaborative efforts can pay substantial dividends. In our partnerships, the American Cancer Society will work in concert with any organization that meets our ethical standards, makes decisions based on scientific evidence, and shares our desire to achieve the stated goal of the partnership.

A final lesson we have learned about selecting partners is to limit the number of organizations in any collaboration to a manageable number. It has been our experience that when an alliance grows too large, the number of conflicting ideas results in such extensive compromise that the original mission may lose its meaning and efficacy. Whereas all of the partner organizations have valid, relevant agendas, they may be so diverse that building consensus requires substantial compromise that may affect the scope of the original mission.

Before approaching potential partners, identify the resources your organization brings to the table. For example, one strength of the American Cancer Society is our ability to enable dialogue. Our medical, scientific, and volunteer base allows us to pull a common thread through disparate communities and tap into a multitude of human and informational assets. When approaching potential partners, we are able to present this capacity as a possible advantage to the coalition.

It is also necessary to clearly understand the goal you hope the partnership will achieve and to be able to explain to potential partners how you can work together to achieve it. It may be wise for each prospective member of the effort to assess the needs of the organization to determine definitively that it will benefit from the association. When groups agree to join the effort, they should immediately establish a clear understanding of the group's mission and commit to working in concert toward it. A written agreement helps the group avoid confusion or conflict in the future. Immediately after building consensus around the goals, define and agree on an equitable division of responsibilities and financing and an impartial system for leadership and governance.

Once the coalition is established, equality is the key to maintaining it. Each partner must be willing to stand down and serve as equals. Every organization must feel that it adds value to the group. Each contributes in a different way, but every contribution must be equally valued. Partners are most effective when they feel that they are each contributing and benefiting equally from the relationship.

This equality is easier to maintain if the group reflects strong individual relationships and strong organizational relationships. The collaboration will be most successful if each partnering organization is represented by an individual who is deeply committed to the group's goals and objectives. These partners must suppress their personal egos and agendas for the good of the group and focus exclusively on the desired outcome.

With different individuals bringing different ideas to the table, the group is likely to encounter some level of tension and conflict. The best way to overcome it and reach consensus is through continual, open communication and interpersonal relationship building. A skilled facilitator may be needed to help keep communication channels open and ensure that all groups' voices are heard equally and to prevent the effort from becoming hobbled by personal differences, conflict, or misunderstandings.

Maintaining this level of communication and equality requires a great deal of flexibility and a commitment to accountability. No member organization should ever compromise its guiding principles, but each should otherwise be prepared to be adaptable. Partners must be held accountable for fulfilling their responsibilities. Coalition leaders should track each group's contributions and keep the entire group continually apprised of progress toward the goal.

Each organization must be willing to commit the resources and people necessary to genuinely help the partnership move forward. Whereas buy-in at the chief executive officer level within each partnering organization is critically important, the effort's true success lies in how deeply rooted the organization's commitment is. The organization with acceptance at multiple levels will be the most successful collaborator.

Finally, and perhaps most important, collaborations require patience. It takes time and energy to break inertia, and whereas an effort may seem ineffective in its first year, it will likely offer a high return on investment in the future that will more than justify the energy and expense. Periodic measurements help keep partners motivated. By continually assessing progress toward the goal and celebrating every victory, partners see that they are making a difference and understand that success will not occur overnight. If all partners are deeply committed to the goal and have a pragmatic expectation of the time frame in which they might realistically achieve it, the effort's momentum will remain strong, and the group will ultimately realize success.

Collaborations work when they share expertise and intellectual collateral. By indulging in the intellectual debate that is a key element of the scientific process, each group in the partnership brings its best thinking forward. This collective wisdom challenges the status quo and helps the effort evolve.

Ultimately, collaborative efforts may make such momentous inroads that the public arena claims ownership of the issue and helps the coalition sustain its momentum. For example, in 1985, cancer control organizations designated the month of October National Breast Cancer Awareness Month (NBCAM) and set about raising public awareness of the disease. These groups' concerted efforts have been so successful that NBCAM is now an international phenomenon that the public has embraced with energy and enthusiasm. If public health organizations stopped hosting NBCAM activities, the effort would likely be sustained through public support alone. This level of public awareness and support is the ultimate measure of success for a collaborative public health effort.

Future of Collaboration

Through collaboration, the American Cancer Society has made significantly more progress toward its mission of eliminating cancer as a major health problem than we could have made alone. We have embraced collaboration as an organizational priority, and it has brought the achievement of our mission within our grasp. We continue to nurture and maintain our existing collaborative relationships while continually seeking new opportunities.

Our Preventive Health Partnership—an alliance with the American Heart Association and the American Diabetes Association—has enhanced our already-substantial collaborative efforts. This unprecedented partnership of traditionally competitive organizations is a unique opportunity to reach more people than ever with the simple message that adhering to many of the same lifestyle factors (controlling weight, quitting smoking, and regular medical care) can greatly reduce risk for all three diseases.

By uniting disparate support bases, our three organizations each reach a much deeper demographic and will therefore be more successful in effecting behavior change that will substantially reduce the number of people affected by cancer, heart disease, and diabetes. By establishing the interconnectedness of these three deadly diseases, the partnership will be far more influential with constituents. This collaboration's potential for saving lives is far greater than any one of the three partners could have achieved singly. The lessons we have learned through successful previous collaborations will guide us through this pioneering, lifesaving partnership.

Conclusion

Since cholera ravaged London in 1849 and a simple pump handle quashed an epidemic, the issues facing public health practitioners have grown increasingly complex, but the challenges are not insurmountable. They simply require a broader mind-set. Human beings are social creatures; if our species thrives on social interaction, it follows that our public health organizations would flourish through collaboration.

No one organization can eradicate the health scourges of the twenty-first century on its own. But by working in tandem with other groups and leveraging each other's strengths to achieve maximum benefit, we can ensure better health and a higher quality of life for all.

References

DeSalle, R. "Solving the Riddle of Cholera Through Medical Geography." In R. DeSalle (ed.), *Epidemic: The World of Infectious Diseases*. New York: American Museum of Natural History, 1999.

Gillies, P. "Effectiveness of Alliances and Partnerships for Health Promotion." *Health Promotion International*, 1998, *13*(2), 99–117.

Shultz, J. *Democracy Owners Manual*. Piscataway, N.J.: Rutgers University Press, 2001.

Part IV

. . . .

Learning from Experience and Building a Generation of Leaders

12

· ·

Leadership Development
for Global Health

Jo Ivey Boufford

There is no doubt that today we are at the cutting edge of scientific and medical advancement. More than ever, we have the knowledge, the tools, and the resources to promote health, prevent illness, and fight disease. Global communication has and will continue to facilitate the immediate transmission of vital information. Health is now a powerful political platform and, more than ever, it is recognized to be central to sustainable economic development (Sachs, 2002).

Despite these facts, each year more than half a million women die of preventable causes during pregnancy and childbirth. This is unacceptable. Health infrastructures in the poorest countries are not well developed, and there are large underserved population groups where priority health needs are unmet. This is unacceptable. Vitamin deficiencies, malnutrition, infectious diseases, and anemia are widespread health issues affecting large portions of the populations of the developing world despite food surpluses, available technology, and scientific breakthroughs. This also is unacceptable. New challenges of chronic disease, mental health, and accidents and injuries will require action.

This chapter draws on research and interviews conducted by the author with support from the Bill and Melinda Gates Foundation during 2003.

In view of the multitude of activities that have already been undertaken, what does make a difference and achieve results? There is evidence that one critical reason for this "implementation gap" at the national health policy and program level is inadequate attention to and investment in the people who must make the health system work and, among them, those who manage and lead it. At the global level, health leaders are missing from critical global policy debates like those on finance, trade, economic development, and agriculture policy that dramatically affect human health. Experienced leaders from the developing world are not equitably represented in global-level health policymaking. If we are to achieve sustainable improvements in global health, as the world community mobilizes to reach the Millennium Development Goals (MDGs), we must pay special attention to the health of Africa, the only region of the world that is moving in the wrong direction on all MDG health indicators. Addressing these issues must be a priority in any strategy to strengthen global health leadership.

Human Resources for Health Systems

It is hard to imagine any activity in the health sector that is not somehow dependent on people, but the topic of human resources for health has been largely neglected. The Rockefeller Foundation has launched a major global Joint Learning Initiative (JLI) to address this gap because "unless we focus on the human component of health systems development, it seems fair to predict that the goals of the global health community such as more equitable access to life saving vaccines and treatments, and the larger scale improvements reflected in the United Nations Millennium Development Goals will not be met" (Rockefeller Foundation, 2003).

Supported by multiple donors, the JLI project operates through seven working groups with global representation, including multilateral and bilateral donors and foundations. The work of the JLI to date has raised overall awareness of the central importance of human resources for health among policymakers at national and global levels and also donors. The recommendations in the final report, due by the end of 2004, should help country-level and global agency leaders develop more robust human resource plans and programs to strengthen the health sector workforce.

There are enormous unmet needs for work in the area of human capacity building for health at the country level and globally to address the adequacy of numbers, types, training, location, and retention of formal and informal health workers, especially to meet the needs of the developing world to deliver personal and population-oriented health services (Leppo, 2001a; World Health Organization, 2000). The World Bank has recently acknowledged its failure to address investments in human resources development for health systems, and new leadership in the health and development sector at the World Bank is committed to addressing this gap in its loan and grants programs (Jacques Badouy of World Bank at World Bank meeting on Human Resources for Health, Oct. 28, 2004).

The World Health Organization (WHO) is working closely with the JLI. In 2000, it was charged by member states (World Health Assembly session 43/Executive Board session 44) to create a human resources development initiative in service of an urgent need to develop sustainable health systems. As part of its human resources for health initiative, WHO commissioned a series of papers and consultations with senior health systems leaders on priority needs for effective and sustainable health systems. The results of an extensive literature review (Leppo, 2001b) and broad consultation were the identification of huge gaps between capacity and the need for leadership in strategic management and policy development at the country level, especially in developing countries and particularly Africa (Milen, 2001). The report called on WHO to mount a major initiative to strengthen its own capacity at central, regional, and country levels to assist countries in these efforts. To reflect its increased emphasis on human health resources, the function has recently been elevated to the departmental level.

Donor support is key to moving any such agenda. At the request of WHO, Glenngård and Anell (2003) attempted to gather data through literature reviews and direct interviews of key leaders in the U.S. Agency for International Development (USAID), the World Bank, Swedish International Development Agency (SIDA), Department for International Development (UK) (DfID), Norwegian Agency for International Development (NORAD), and Danish International Development Agency (DANIDA) on the kinds and amounts of donor investment in human resources development for health and, within that category, leadership development. Only SIDA was able to identify specific budgets for the support of such programs because most are integrated with overall project budgets. It was not possible to break out specific programs on leadership development in this work. In other literature of international programs, there is little documented evidence of investment in leadership development for broader health systems effectiveness and virtually none on leadership for global health.

Their data do show that most donor support is for short-term education and training to address shortages and imbalances in technical areas or to staff vertical programs. A shift has been occurring from donor-driven programs to those owned, developed, and managed by the recipient countries, but the recent surge in funding for disease-specific programs such as provision of antiretroviral therapy for patients infected with human immunodeficiency virus (HIV) or with the acquired immunodeficiency syndrome (AIDS), tuberculosis treatment, and so on may reverse this trend. Such programs have tended to focus on front-line workers, with little explicit investment to address the overall human resources issues or the specific management and leadership gaps in the health systems of the developing countries with the greatest disease burden.

Need for Leadership Development for Health Systems and Global Health

Leadership development should be supported not for its own sake but because it contributes to the achievement of a goal—in this case, improvements in country-level health systems and global health.

There is evidence that leadership action for improved global health is required at three levels of governance and organization: at the national level for in-country action, at the regional level where groups of countries work together, and in the supranational and global organizations that affect health. Leaders at each level must be able to use evidence to advocate for the policies and resources needed. And they must be able to cross boundaries to work across the different levels of government and with individuals and organizations outside the health sector that have enormous influence on health decision making like those in finance, trade, education, environment, and economic development.

Leadership at Country Level

Many articles and reports discuss the need for individuals who possess knowledge and skills commonly associated in the literature with leadership. The Commission on Macroeconomics and Health calls for the building of country capacity for stewardship, intersectoral action, and monitoring of performance (Sachs, 2002). The New Partnership for African Development (Buch, 2003) speaks to the same concerns as does the World Development Report 2003 (World Bank, 2003). Mills, Bennett, and Russell (2001) call for individuals with the skills to manage change, address organizational cultures, and cope with external constraints. A significant number of experts I interviewed to explore the needs for global health leadership over the past year called for improved country-level leadership for health within all sectors (government, civil society, and business) working together to increase the effectiveness of current vertical programs and to strengthen health systems.

The effectiveness of individual leaders is closely related to the availability of institutional support for their efforts. Because institutions are often weak, the leaders that do exist, especially in developing countries, have great difficulty implementing viable solutions that would make a difference in the health of their population.

This is due to a variety of factors, but among those that were considered, expert advisors considered the following to be most crucial:

- Rapid turnover of leadership, interrupting prior agendas

- The failure to create the context surrounding health leaders that would enable them to devise and implement strategies to achieve their goals, including

     the lack of access to up-to-date knowledge and technology

     the lack of capacity to collect and present convincing evidence on the health situation at the national level that would enable them to make the case for resources among competing priorities

     donor-driven agendas that alter national priorities, are short term, and fail to build sustainable health systems

- The lack of sustainable institutional mechanisms that enable potential leaders to draw on the wealth of expertise at the country, regional, or global level, including

     the lack of alliances with critical groups—for example, politicians, consumer groups, academia, nongovernmental organizations (NGOs), and so on

     the lack of understanding of and involvement in issues of a global nature that affect health at the

country level—for example, global financial decisions, treaties, trade, commerce, and so on

These factors have prevented effective, sustained leadership for
health, especially from countries of the South that could have contributed significantly to the unfinished global health agenda.

It takes leadership, individual and institutional, to develop the
evidence of need, design effective interventions, create effective
policies, argue for resources, mobilize the public and political will
to act for health, and address inequities globally and within countries. It takes effective leadership to create a vision for an effective
health system and to negotiate effectively with donors and funding
agencies. It takes effective leadership to coordinate and integrate
what may be disparate vertical programs into an effective and flexible health system capable of responding to crisis and meeting basic
needs. It is this leadership that can make a difference within countries and at a global level.

Leadership at Global Level

A more recent influence on country-level health progress is the
issue of globalization. The following key factors of globalization
influence health:

- People flow: travel, migration (forced and voluntary),
  patient movement, movement of health workers

- Information flow: ideas and popular culture, commercial health information, health education, scientific or
  medical evidence

- Technology: information and electronic technologies
  and direct telemedicine links, biomedical and scientific
  technologies

- Commerce: movements of goods and services, regulatory frameworks (food, drug, and blood quality; health

care standards setting; intellectual property), and capital markets (including trade policy)

- Environment

- Diseases

- Wars, violence, and crime

- Religion and culture

The effects of globalization are superimposed on the national factors influencing health. For example, international trade policy affects food safety and the availability of pharmaceuticals; a global labor market contributes to the migration of key health professionals from developing countries to the developed. These are all factors outside the exclusive control of nation-states. The consequences of decisions made at the global level, especially those related to trade and commerce, often escape health leaders at global and national levels. In the absence of strong health leadership, ministers of finance and heads of state make decisions at the country level and in global forums without being aware of their health consequences.

Several authors have identified the need for stronger national leadership on global health issues. It is needed to make country-level health systems more effective in the face of global determinants of health (Kaul, Grunberg, and Stern, 1999; Feacham, 2001) to create the ability to take the "outside" into account. Strong leadership is also needed to ensure that the health effects of global initiatives are clear and that these respond more effectively to country needs (Sachs, 2002; Chen, Evans, and Cash, 1999; McKee, Garner, and Stott, 2001; Mills, 2002).

Kaul, Grunberg, and Stern (1999) identify three gaps in public policymaking that inhibit the sharing of global public goods: one of these is the "participation gap" in which global policymaking is essentially intergovernmental but some governments (especially those of countries in the South) are not represented or, if present, do not have the capacity either to participate fully or follow up effectively on commitments made because of a lack of experience, resources, or power.

Rao (1999) and Stiglitz (1999) both agree on the problems of global governance being dominated by wealthy industrial countries and the equity issues this raises. Mills (2002) calls for a "leveling of the playing field" to create a global partnership based on shared responsibility and mutual interest. Buse, Drayer, Fustkian, and Lee (2002) caution that absent this level playing field, there may be a false policy convergence due to inequities in power of those at the table. They provide a case study of a recent global health debate dominated by a "transnational managerial class" of U.S. consulting firms, multilateral donors, foundations, WHO, and private-sector interests—a phenomenon they call "elite pluralism." Many of those interviewed stressed the importance of better preparation and linkage of leaders in developing countries with global decision making to put them on a more equal power footing.

A Model for Leadership Development

There is no agreed-on definition of "leadership." Larson and others (2002) cite more than three hundred different definitions in the literature. Much of this variation is because of the increasing understanding that leadership occurs in context and that organizations increasingly prefer to create their own definition to fit their strategy and culture. The literature on leadership and approaches to leadership development is voluminous. (For example, a bibliography on collaborative leadership, a currently popular approach, commissioned by the Turning Point Leadership Development National Excellence Collaborative in the United States [Larson and others, 2002], identified nearly three hundred thousand citations on "collaborative leadership in public health." About thirty-five thousand were reviewed for their project.)

In health, the word "leadership" is attached to programs ranging from short courses in a specific disease or other technical area to graduate-degree-granting fellowships to midcareer and "in-practice" executive programs. Most sponsors seem to use the term to imply that anyone who participates in "their" program will, by definition, be a leader. To some degree, the prestige, the kinds of exposures outside a person's experience, or increased knowledge and skills from a course or receipt of a degree may put them in a leadership position back in their home environments. However, the actual time spent specific to the leadership development process varies considerably, if present at all, and the contribution of the program to participants' leadership effectiveness is rarely measured.

The public health community in the United States, led by the Centers for Disease Control and Prevention, has long supported investments in public health "systems" leadership development in the United States through the National Public Health Leadership Institute, now at the University of North Carolina, and internationally through its own Sustainable Management Development Program. The Epidemiologic Intelligence Service and its international counterpart, the Field Epidemiology Training Program (FETP), produce elite technical cadres of leaders for public health. However, a recent evaluation of FETP makes the point that when these programs fail, they almost always fail because of lack of leadership skills and team building. In recent years, more content has been added on leadership to the FETP programs adapted to the specific country context (Setliff and others, 2003).

In the international arena, the Fogarty Center at the National Institutes of Health has a long history in the area of international leadership development for biomedical research, and they have recently extended this work into areas of epidemiology and clinical research. They also emphasize the importance of leadership abilities to fellows' success when they return to their countries and the need for explicit financial support in the form of "return grants"

(Gerald Keusch, director of the Fogarty Center, National Institutes of Health, interview, Nov. 18, 2003).

Leadership development is a major focus of the top Fortune 500 companies. Melum (2002) notes that leadership development is big business. In 1993, U.S. companies spent $17 billion annually to develop leadership skills in their staff. The health care industry has been slow to invest in leadership, spending about 1.25 percent of payroll on overall training and leadership development each year compared with 4 percent in the top one hundred companies in 2002.

Chief Executive magazine (Spiro, 2003), in cooperation with Hewitt Associates (a global human resources firm), annually ranks the top twenty companies for leadership development. Criteria include self-reported data gathered by Hewitt from the firms, financial performance data, and the judgment of an external panel of experts from business and academia. Johnson and Johnson, IBM, and General Electric are the top three. Their approaches vary depending on their corporate culture, structure (centralized versus decentralized), and strategy. But they all emphasize growing their own top leaders and supporting up-and-comers. Most develop their own list of preferred leadership qualities, even definitions of leadership, to match their strategy and culture and train to those. Webster (2003) writes of companies in the developing world that see leadership as a critical risk factor in global success. She also notes the importance of an organizational culture that supports the use of the techniques learned by leaders.

Calculating the effects and the return on investment in leadership development is an issue critical to institutions across the public, nonprofit, and corporate spectrum. Anecdotal information abounds in the business sector, but it has been a challenge for them to develop quantitative measurement tools. Most of the work done on returns on investment and benefit-cost ratios has looked at different types of training not specifically called leadership development. The studies done have tended to focus on employee groups (supervisors) whose work can be directly related to financial returns. Phillips (1996) notes studies of supervisor or manager training with returns on investment of 400 percent (benefit-cost ratio of 5:1), 215 percent (benefit-cost ratio, 3:1), and 1,400 percent (benefit-cost ratio, 15:1).

Phillips has developed the most sophisticated model to date for evaluating return on investment. It requires data collection at five levels: participant reaction and plans to use training, demonstrated learning, applied learning on the job, did on-the-job application produce measurable results, and did the monetary value of the returns exceed the cost of the training. He discusses the challenges of gathering good data on each, especially the last item. When financial outcome is less relevant than social outcome, the metrics are even more challenging.

A report from the Office of Public Management (2003) traces the evolution of thinking in the general literature on leadership theory and practice and its importance to organizational change. Moving from the "great man theory" of the mid-twentieth century to the more current notions of collaborative leadership, the challenge now is to strengthen and mobilize the leadership potential of all actors in an organization to work with their collaborators outside to achieve a defined goal.

There is, however, an emerging agreement in the health, development (Office of Public Management, 2003; David and Lucille Packard Foundation Population Program, 2000; Leadership Learning Community, 2003; Neufeld and Johnson, 2004), and business literature that working with individuals already in positions of authority and responsibility leads to faster results. There is also agreement that the characteristics of effective leadership development programs at this level include

- Programs built around the process of solving the actual problems faced by participants (leadership for what?)

- Programs that develop the personal and professional leadership skills of participants

- Programs sensitive to the real environments (advantages and constraints) in which the participants operate

- Models involving several short-term engagements with brief outside exposures over a twelve- to eighteen-month period, interspersed with specific commitments to on-site project work and support at the home site

- A cohort model providing the opportunity for peer learning during and after the program

- A team experience or approach

- Mentoring or technical assistance (or both) in the longer term to support participants' efforts at organizational change

- Long-term continuity of support through coaching, peer networking, resource sharing, and periodic reunions to permit reflection on learning

Leadership programs for global health should also include the following:

- Formal content on globalization and its effects on health

- Exposure to and understanding of the key global organizations affecting health and health policy

- Attention to the skills needed to work across cultural, organizational, and governmental boundaries at national, regional, and global levels

- Programs that involve individuals from multiple sectors, not only health professionals

- Priority given to leadership development for those
  from countries carrying the highest burden of disease
  to prepare them for active participation in global
  policymaking

It is also critically important that individuals from participating countries are partners in the design of the leadership development program to assure that it is relevant to the challenges they face and the resources they have to meet them.

Taking into consideration the literature, experience, and expert advice in the area of leadership development to achieve results most quickly for global health, major investments are needed in practice-based leadership development for certain key groups of individuals currently in (or likely to be in the future) positions of authority and responsibility for achieving better health outcomes at the national level and in global organizations. The goal of these programs would be to increase individuals' effectiveness in their current roles, strengthen their organizations, and prepare them for global health leadership.

The model below developed by the Office of Public Management (Office of Public Management, 2003) (see Figure 12.1) provides the conceptual framework for such an approach. Individuals enter the program with different personal qualities, knowledge, skills, and experience. Through specific learning modules, including structured lectures and discussions with experts, readings, case studies (including technical content as appropriate), study visits, and peer learning, they increase their self-awareness, learn to broaden their behavioral repertoire and build good-quality relationships, and develop and articulate a vision for stronger health systems and improved health results. This vision will guide the formulation of a leadership agenda that is uniquely suited to the environment in which they work. Their ability to analyze this environment, organizational and political, will be strengthened along with their strategic judgment that must consider local and also national and global

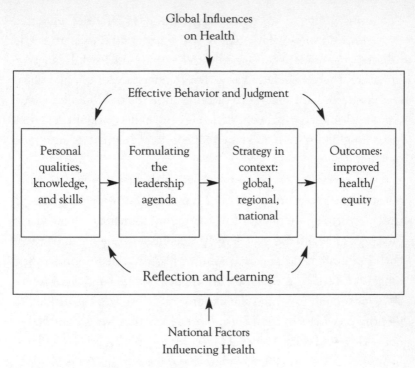

Figure 12.1. A Model of Leadership Development

influences. They learn to mobilize others to work for the defined goals, including the development of leadership capacity of others in the organization to achieve and sustain the identified outcome. Mentorship and peer learning during and after the formal program permit reflection on their work and modification of their strategy and actions.

Next Steps

In their article *Leadership for Global Health*, the Office of Public Management (2003) investigated multiple sources to identify existing leadership development programs for global health for the target groups and including the program elements outlined above. After examining literature and written descriptions of offerings supported by current donors, WHO, the World Bank, and universities and regional organizations concerned with health in the English-language literature, there were few, if any, that included experiential, midcareer programs with strong attention to individual skill building and organizational context; generic leadership skills or qualities; and a focus on globalization and its effects on health at the country and regional levels.

A large number of providers in the North offer the first two without specific linkage to health or, if they are health-related, focus on the domestic challenges of the particular country. Others with a more global health focus are largely didactic or academic in content, with little focus on personal and professional development and longer-term support. Because they are personalized and labor intensive, most such programs are expensive. More work is needed to identify providers in the South, but the few that were identified in our review and those identified in work for the JLI by Neufeld and Johnson (2004) have an academic base, often business schools, and offer degree or executive development programs, but the target group is not clear. There are also some NGOs, especially those in reproductive health that have historically offered a strong training component in that field that are beginning to offer training to other groups, but not yet at the level of systems leadership or global focus needed, largely because of a lack of experience and resources.

As attention to and investment in human resources for health at the country and global levels increase, the role of leadership must be an important part of whatever initiatives are developed.

The evidence for the critical role leadership plays in closing the implementation gap in policy and programming for country-level and global health is clear. It is important that those in positions of responsibility at national and global agency levels see the value in continuing to develop their own leadership capabilities and that of those around them. It is important that they know that the expertise exists to make them more effective and that taking advantage of it is not a sign of weakness but a normal part of a leader's responsibility in such a complex and changing world. This conversation must begin to be common within global and regional organizations where health leaders come together and among donors as they consider their funding strategies to improve global health.

Key to these efforts to enrich the quality of global health decision making are individuals in developing countries and those in transition who have or will soon have the responsibility for health systems leadership in their own countries and those who will play a role at the global level in health policymaking within global health organizations and in broader policy forums. A major priority of these development efforts should be in Africa, which bears the greatest disease burden.

Significant resources will be needed over the long term. Action might also be accelerated by an explicit project to heighten awareness of the importance of leadership and the fact that available expertise can be harnessed to develop additional capacity.

Important activities to pursue a leadership development agenda for global health should include the following:

- The identification of providers of high-level experience-based leadership development programs worldwide in health and other sectors that may be applicable

- The creation and maintenance of a learning network of these providers to share experiences, approaches, and the results of their programs to date

- A process to determine the needs for leadership development within the key health and health-related global agencies and with interested country-level health leaders, especially in the South

- Programs to use existing provider resources to build the capacity of existing or new organizations to provide high-level leadership development that is relevant and responsive to the needs of global agencies and developing countries, especially those in Africa

• The establishment of an evidence base on leadership development strategies and methods through both documentation and evaluation of these efforts to inform the future design of country-level, regional, and global agency programs

Such an effort will be most productive if well coordinated and linked to key global organizations like WHO or the World Bank Institute. It could be a time-limited project conducted by consultants during its exploratory phase, but as this phase yields learning about availability and demand, a more formal structure would more likely assure progress on this critical agenda. WHO has also proposed a series of centers of excellence for human resource development in key regions of the world; such an effort could include a focal point on leadership development to distinguish it from the necessary development of managerial and human resources expertise.

There undoubtedly are many approaches to moving the leadership development agenda, but the timing is urgent if we are to fulfill the promise of effectively applying our knowledge to make a difference for global health, especially in the countries in greatest need.

References

Buch, E. *The New Partnership for Africa's Development Health Strategy: Initial Program of Action*. Pretoria, South Africa: University of Pretoria, New Partnership for Africa's Development, 2003.

Buse, K., Drayer, N., Fustkian, S., and Lee, K. "Globalization and Health Policy: Terms and Opportunity." In K. Lee, K. Buse, and S. Fustkian (eds.), *Health Policy in a Globalising World*. Cambridge, U.K.: Cambridge University Press, 2002, Chap. 14.

Chen, L. C., Evans, T. G., and Cash, R. A. "Health as a Global Public Good." In I. Kaul, I. Grunberg, and M. A. Stern (eds.), *Global Public Goods: International Cooperation in the 21st Century*. New York: Oxford University Press, 1999.

David and Lucille Packard Foundation Population Program. *Future Leaders: Programmatic Directions*. Los Altos, Calif.: David and Lucille Packard Foundation, 2000.

Feacham, R.G.A. "The Role of Governments." In C. E. Koop, C. Pearson, and M. R. Schwarz (eds.), *Critical Issues in Global Health*. San Francisco: Jossey-Bass, 2001, Chap. 4.

Glenngård, A., and Anell, A. *Investment in Human Resources for Health: Problems, Approaches, and Donor Experiences*. Lund: Swedish Institute for Health Economics, 2003.

Kaul, I., Grunberg, I., and Stern, M. A. (eds.). *Global Public Goods: International Cooperation in the 21st Century*. New York: Oxford University Press, 1999.

Larson, C., and others (eds.). *Collaborative Leadership and Health: A Review of the Literature*. Seattle: Turning Point National Program Office, University of Washington, 2002.

Leadership Learning Community. "Leadership Development Programs: Investment in Individuals." New York: Ford Foundation, Leadership Learning Community, 2003. Available: http://www.grantcraft.org.

Leppo, K. *Governing and Managing Health Systems: Scaling Up Strategic Capacities in Countries*. Geneva: World Health Organization, 2001a.

Leppo, K. *Strengthening Capacities for Policy Development: Strategic Management in National Health Systems*. Geneva: World Health Organization, 2001b.

McKee, M., Garner, P., and Stott, R. *International Cooperation in Health*. Oxford, U.K.: Oxford University Press, 2001.

Melum, M. "Developing High Performance Leaders." *Quality Management in Health Care*, 2002, 2(1), 55–68.

Milen, A. *What Do We Know About Capacity Building: An Overview of Existing Knowledge and Good Practice*. Geneva: World Health Organization, 2001.

Mills, A., Bennett, S., and Russell, S. *The Challenges of Health Sector Reform: What Must Governments Do?* New York: Palgrave, 2001.

Mills, G. *Poverty to Prosperity: Globalization, Good Governance, and African Recovery*. Johannesburg and Cape Town: South African Institute of International Affairs and Tafelburg Publishers, 2002.

Neufeld, V., and Johnson, N. "Training and Development of Leaders." Paper commissioned for the Joint Learning Initiative, Rockefeller Foundation, New York, Feb. 2004.

Office of Public Management. *Leadership for Global Health*. London: Office of Public Management, 2003.

Phillips, J. "ROI: The Search for Best Practices." *Training and Development*, 1996, 50(2), 42–47.

Rao, M. "Equity in a Global Public Framework." In I. Kaul, I. Grunberg, and M. A. Stern (eds.), *Global Public Goods: International Cooperation in the 21st Century*. New York: Oxford University Press, 1999, pp. 68–87.

Rockefeller Foundation. *Human Resources for Health and Development: A Joint Learning Initiative*. New York: Rockefeller Foundation, 2003.

Sachs, J. (ed.). *Commission on Macroeconomics and Health*. Geneva: World Health Organization, 2002.

Setliff, R., and others. "Strengthening the Public Health Workforce: Three CDC Programs That Prepare Managers and Leadership for the Challenges of the 21st Century." *Journal of Public Health Management and Practice*, 2003, 9(2), 91–102.

Spiro, L. N. "In Search of Leaders." *Chief Executive Magazine*, Oct. 2003, p. 192.

Stiglitz, J. E. "Knowledge as a Global Public Good." In I. Kaul, I. Grunberg, and M. A. Stern (eds.), *Global Public Goods: International Cooperation in the 21st Century*. New York: Oxford University Press, 1999, pp. 308–325.

Webster, E. "Successful Companies Link Leadership, Future Strategy." *Business Day [South Africa]*, Oct. 2003, p. 14.

World Bank. "Sustainable Development in a Dynamic World: Transforming Institutions, Growth, and Quality of Life." *World Development Report 2003*. Washington, D.C.: International Bank for Reconstruction and Development, World Bank, 2003.

World Health Organization. "Health Systems: Improving Performance." *World Health Report 2000*. Geneva: World Health Organization, 2000.

13

Challenges to Health in Eastern Europe
and the Former Soviet Union

A Decade of Experience

Martin McKee

Largely unrecognized by the rest of the world, a health catastrophe was slowly unfolding in the Soviet Union and its satellites from the 1960s onward. At a time when life expectancy was increasing rapidly in Western Europe, it was initially stagnating and then, in the countries emerging from the Soviet Union, falling rapidly: by 1994, male life expectancy at birth in Russia had declined to less than fifty-eight years, a decrease since 1987 of more than seven years (McKee, 2001). Yet, these aggregate figures concealed the true scale of the problem. Unlike the situation in many developing and middle-income countries, infant and child mortality is relatively low and has been falling continuously. In this region, it was the high adult mortality, especially among men, that was driving the crisis, with the leading causes being injuries, violence, and cardiovascular diseases (Walberg and others, 1998). And although women appeared

It is impossible to mention all the people who have made possible the achievements described in this chapter. However, a few deserve special mention. They include, in addition to those mentioned in the text, Nina Schwalbe and Noah Simmons at the Open Society Institute; Dineke Zeegers-Paget at the European Public Health Association; Thierry Louvet at the Association of Schools of Public Health in the European Region; Tom Novotny, formerly at the World Bank; Lenart Kohler at the Nordic School of Public Health; Dan Enachescu in Bucharest; and Vilius Grabauskas in Kaunas. I also thank my colleagues at the London School of Hygiene and Tropical Medicine who, individually and collectively, have done so much to support the development of public health in this region.

to be faring better, in terms of mortality, they, too, were suffering from high levels of poor self-rated health and thus levels of healthy life expectancy that are similar to men (Andreev, McKee, and Shkolnikov, forthcoming).

These events were taking place in countries that had until recently been part of one of the world's two superpowers. The Soviet Union could arm itself with sufficient nuclear warheads to destroy humanity, but its successor countries were unable to prevent the premature deaths of thousands of their citizens from entirely avoidable causes. Their earlier achievements, in particular the control of major communicable diseases such as diphtheria and tuberculosis, were being reversed. And worse was to come, as the human immunodeficiency virus (HIV) began to spread into a population with few prospects who were increasingly taking solace in the use of intravenous drugs; the former Soviet Union is experiencing the fastest rise in cases of acquired immunodeficiency syndrome (AIDS) anywhere in the world (Hamers and Downs, 2003).

The outlook was not so pessimistic everywhere. Some countries of Central and Eastern Europe experienced improved health soon after the political transition (Zatonski, McMichael, and Powles, 1998; Dolea, Nolte, and McKee, 2002). In the three Baltic States, life expectancy followed a trajectory that was, despite their new-found independence, remarkably similar to that in Russia until 1998 when they at last began to diverge as the Russian currency crisis of that year was followed by a further decline in life expectancy. In the Baltic republics, it continued upward, albeit at a level still well behind that in their Western neighbors; on current trends, they will not converge until 2032.

In summary, whereas life expectancy in Central Europe is at last improving, although more slowly than is desirable, many countries of the former Soviet Union share the unwanted distinction, with sub-Saharan Africa, of actually experiencing a reversal in life expectancy (McMichael, McKee, Shkolnikov, and Valkonen, 2002). In all of these settings, a new generation of strong and effective leaders who can be advocates for healthy public policies is clearly needed. In this chapter, I review the progress that has been made so far in supporting their development.

Legacy of the Past

Any consideration of health policy in the former Communist bloc cannot ignore the legacy of the past. The Communist bloc can be divided into those countries that were part of the Soviet Union before World War II and those that had Communism imposed on them after 1945. Of course, there was diversity within these two groupings, and a few countries (Albania, Yugoslavia, and Mongolia) needed to be considered separately.

Although scientists in many of the Communist countries in Central Europe, such as Hungary and Poland, were able to participate in international scientific networks and worked within a scientific paradigm that was little different from that in the West, the environment in which scientific debate took place in the Soviet Union had many similarities with Europe in the years before the Renaissance. This fact is less well recognized than it should be, and its influence remains a factor to be taken into account even now.

Understanding Soviet Science

Copernicus and Vesalius confronted a world in which the writings of ancient authorities, in their cases Ptolemy and Galen, had ultimate authority (Gribbin, 2003). Similarly, in the Soviet Union, scientists were expected to show how their interpretations were consistent with their disciplinary founding fathers (*osnovopolozhnik*), such as Michurin in biology or Pavlov in psychology, or better, to the ideological founders of Communism, Marx, Engels, Lenin, and Stalin (Krementosov, 1997). This led to the obligatory use of what were termed "nomadic quotations," with sayings of great men being used to justify whatever was being argued, however tenuous the connection. The researcher was assisted by compilations of quotations, as in a book published in 1936 that stated confidently how "there is not a single principal problem in modern biology, the approach to the solution of which has not been pointed out by the founders of Marxism" (Tokin and others, 1936).

The Soviet Union also resembled the early Renaissance in Western Europe because scientific debate was settled on the basis of ideological (previously religious) authority. Finally, both systems were willing to impose the ultimate penalty for dissent from the official line, be they Giordano Bruno, burned in 1600 for espousing the ideas of Copernicus, or Nikolai Vavilov, the leading Soviet geneticist who challenged the prevailing orthodoxy and died in the Gulag in 1943 (Soyfer, 2001).

In a society where a hint of contact with the West could lead to a long period of imprisonment or worse, with extremely limited access to international scientific literature, it was unsurprising that a distinctive scientific paradigm emerged. Perhaps the best-known manifestation was the ascendancy of Trofin Lysenko, a Ukrainian agriculturalist who rejected mendelian ideas, arguing that intergenerational change in plants arose from adaptation to changing circumstances (Joravsky, 1970). His influence on Soviet agriculture was disastrous but, despite accumulating evidence of the failure of his theories, he survived for many years because of the high-level political support he received. Yet, there were many similar examples in other areas, such as Olga Lepeshinskkaia, who argued for a pre-Pasteurian idea of spontaneous generation of microorganisms from noncellular matter (Krementosov, 1997), or the considerable literature on the effects of sunspot cycles on a wide variety of health outcomes, a literature that owes more to astrology than science.

This environment was hostile to developing either an understanding of the causes of the health crisis that was emerging or the interventions that might effectively respond to it (Field, 1990). This weakness went all the way from individual to population-based interventions. Thus, Soviet medicine gave great prominence to unevaluated methods of treatment that were often based on the application of physical forces, such as magnetism, electric fields, ultraviolet light, or hyperbaric therapy. These also had the advantages of being relatively cheap and easily available in a society where the distribution system was extremely unreliable. They also fit with a prevailing medical model: individuals were not trusted to take responsibility for their own health, and as a consequence, anyone requiring a course of treatment would be admitted to hospital to be sure they took it. In these circumstances, it is unsurprising that when deaths from causes amenable to health care were falling steadily in the West, they remained stubbornly high in the Soviet Union (Andreev and others, 2003).

The medicalization of health was also apparent in population-based interventions. Thus, concepts of social marketing of health were unknown, and behavioral change was expected to arise from mass educational campaigns. Many activities labeled as "prevention" involved widespread and largely ineffective population screening programs. Although such activities were also common in the West until the 1950s, only now have they declined in use in many parts of the former Soviet Union as a consequence of resource constraints in the 1990s. A review of the Russian-language literature, conducted in the late 1990s on causes of the health crisis facing the former Soviet Union, showed how rarely the by-then-considerable research on this topic that had been published in the international literature was cited by leading Russian academics (Tkatchenko, McKee, and Tsouros, 2000). However, there were a few exceptions: in the 1980s, some scientists were permitted to participate in some international networks, largely under the auspices of the World Health Organization (WHO), such as the MONICA program to monitor trends in cardiovascular disease (Tunstall-Pedoe and others, 1999). The Baltic republics were more open than others, for example, participating in the Kaunas-Rotterdam study of heart disease (Bosma and others, 1994), but in general, the opportunities to look outside the Soviet Union were limited.

Even if the nature of the problem and the potential remedies had been understood, there was little that could have been done. A rigid system of command and control, with all aspects of an individual's life ordered according to central *diktats*, provided little room for innovation. Again, there were a few places where individuals did overcome these problems and develop effective, mostly small-scale programs, but these were rare.

Central and Eastern Europe

It has already been noted that the situation was different in most of the countries of Central and Eastern Europe outside the Soviet Union, where scientists could interact relatively freely with their counterparts in the West, although there were some exceptions. A particularly tragic example is Ceausescu's Romania, where the misguided use of microtransfusions to strengthen undernourished children had the unintended consequence of creating an epidemic of HIV infection (Kozinetz, Matusa, and Cazazu, 2000). Another was Albania, a country long cut off from the rest of Europe by high mountains and malarial marshes, which remained largely untouched by developments such as motorized transport until 1990, secure behind ideological barriers that isolated it from the rest of the Communist bloc (Gjonca, 2001). Yet, even in the more open societies in Central Europe, the prevailing model of public health practice was one based on outdated concepts of "hygiene" (Bojan, McKee, and Ostbye, 1994), and the regimes were largely unable to respond to the worsening health of their populations and, in particular, the increase in adult mortality (Chenet and others, 1996).

There is but one exception: Yugoslavia, a country that although Communist was outside the Soviet bloc. Although political dissent was not tolerated, it was much more open than its northern neighbors. Unlike them, Yugoslavia also had a public health community that was exposed to developments elsewhere and was able to move with the times. An important factor was the existence of a cohort of professionals trained in modern public health, in particular those associated with the Andrija Stampar School of Public Health in Zagreb, Croatia. It was one of the schools of public health established by the Rockefeller Foundation in the 1920s by the founding father of WHO, Andrija Stampar. In the 1970s and 1980s, the school played a major role in the spread of ideas about primary health care internationally (Borovecki, Belicza, and Oreskovic, 2002).

As this brief review shows, therefore, the situation in this region is different from that in many other parts of the world that are facing major threats to health. The problem is not one of basic capacity. The Soviet system trained many health professionals and built many health facilities, even if it failed to maintain them (Healy and McKee, 2002). But it was completely unable to assess health needs and design and implement effective policies that would respond to them (McKee and others, 2000). Those working at the local level, who were best placed to understand the scale and nature of the threats to health, had neither the tools nor the power to do anything about them. Thus, the challenge was not to build something completely new but to reorient what is already there. The experience of doing so will now be examined. This will focus on two examples, the first from Hungary—like other countries in Central and Eastern Europe, one of the early reformers—and the second from Russia, where the economic crisis of the early 1990s and the more difficult path to democracy delayed reform.

Creating a New Generation of Public Health Leaders

During the 1980s, many of the countries of Central and Eastern Europe had individuals who were at least aware of the nature of the health crisis facing their societies and that something could be done about it. As soon as the borders opened, they sought sympathetic individuals in Western countries, leading to fruitful collaborations. In some cases, the initial encounters owed much to chance, such as the availability of funding from a particular Western country to organize a study tour.

There were two immediate problems: one was to reach consensus about what needed to be done, and the other was to build capacity to do it. And much needed to be done. It would be possible to take examples of these activities from different countries in the region, but this would be misleading because, in reality, success was greatest where all the components were closely linked. Hungary is, arguably, the country where this was most successful, and the following section examines its experience in detail.

Development of Modern Public Health in Hungary

In 1990, Hungarians had the worst health in Central Europe; Hungary's public health system, like that of its neighbors, was based on the Soviet model of sanitary-epidemiological centers whose approach was based on inspection, sanctions, and a medicalized model of health education (Bojan and McKee, 1997). Yet, it also had many things in its favor. There was widespread agreement that something had to be done, even if what it should be was less certain, and there was a well-established, informal network of public health professionals. Unlike some of its neighbors, many senior academic staff had trained abroad, although few in modern public health. Perhaps most important, there was Professor Ferenc Bojan, who could provide both inspirational leadership and the ability to get things done.

Differing views about the nature of public health were addressed explicitly. Many county public health offices had little understanding of modern concepts of public health. However, these ideas were understood by others, in particular individuals with a background in sociology, but their lack of a medical training sometimes made it difficult to be listened to in what was still a highly medicalized culture. One problem was that there were seven different words in Hungarian that meant "public health," although some had unfortunate connotations, like the term "hygiene police" might have in English. A consensus conference involving 150 people from a wide range of interests examined differing approaches to public health, including experience from abroad, and led to a consensus statement

(White, Watt, Bojan, and McKee, 1993). The next task was to develop a means for those interested in public health to discuss it. A professional association was created that was multidisciplinary from the outset, providing a model that others soon followed.

It was also necessary to reform public health training. This began with undergraduate medical training. The four Hungarian medical schools formed a consortium with academic departments in the West, funded by the European Union (McKee, Bojan, White, and Ostbye, 1995). This provided infrastructure, such as computers, faxes, and travel, for short courses and exchanges. A common curriculum was agreed on and new educational methods adopted, incorporating problem-based learning and project work (Bojan, Belicza, Horvath, and McKee, 1995). The experience created a strong basis for action when Hungary agreed to a World Bank health sector loan. This funded two new schools—one for public health within the university in Debrecen and the other for health services management within the university in Budapest. It supported master's and doctoral training abroad, creating a critical mass of trained staff. The development of these institutions was coordinated with other elements of the World Bank loan, overseen by an advisory board comprising Hungarian and Western experts.

From the beginning, an international perspective was emphasized, with both schools participating actively at a European level through the Association of Schools of Public Health in the European Region (ASPHER) and the European Public Health Association (EUPHA). However, in 1995, just after the new school of public health opened, Bojan was killed in a traffic accident, a tragic reminder of the human dimension of the mortality statistics in that region.

Under his successor, Professor Roza Adany, the school has prospered, strengthening relations with the university, the public health service, and local government. An advisory board brought together key stakeholders, and a concordat with the public health service required those appointed to senior posts to be trained in public health; the school also expanded its program of continuing education for those in post. The two organizations also established a network of surveillance centers, providing a basis for epidemiological research. Together, they are contributing effectively to public health in Hungary.

Creating a New Generation of Public Health Leaders in Russia

The situation in Russia was different in almost every respect. The health situation was worse than in Hungary and, in the early 1990s, was deteriorating rapidly rather than improving. Hungary was a small country in Central Europe; Russia was the world's largest, stretching from the Baltic Sea to the Pacific Ocean. Few senior people spoke English, restricting their access to the international literature. Many policies were grounded in an antiscientific paradigm. Transparency in decision making and the development of mature democratic institutions were mere aspirations.

As in Hungary, there were people who recognized the need for change. Igor Denisov, vice rector of the Moscow Medical Academy, had been the last Minister of Health of the Soviet Union. He recognized the scale of crisis facing his country and the need to train a new generation to develop and implement the policies to tackle it.

In many ways, Denisov's actions mirrored those in Hungary. A first step involved strategic alliances with Western partners who could provide expertise and unlock funding opportunities, in this case initially with American universities, such as Emory in Atlanta, and with the Hadassah School of Public Health in Jerusalem. It was then necessary to identify training opportunities to create a faculty trained in modern public health. This was facilitated by funding from the Israeli government and the Soros Foundation; a generation of young Russians was trained in Jerusalem under the leadership of Dr. Ted Tulchinsky. A second step was to create a public health network of institutions pursuing similar goals. An informal partnership was developed between the Moscow Medical Academy and academic departments in St. Petersburg, Tver, and Chelyabinsk.

A third step involved links with local communities and national and international agencies.

As in Hungary, an international advisory board was established. Initially, it focused on institutional development but soon became a vehicle for developing further collaboration, such as the United Kingdom Department for International Development's program that funds posts held jointly by the Moscow Medical Academy and the London School of Hygiene and Tropical Medicine.

Other Examples

These are only two of many examples that could have been chosen. Another success story is the BRIMHEALTH program (Kohler and Eklund, 2002), where the Nordic School of Public Health, in partnership with academic departments in Estonia, Latvia, Lithuania, and Russia, has prepared the groundwork for new schools of public health in each of those countries. Graduates are now helping new schools in other ex-Soviet republics, especially in Central Asia (Kalediene, 2002). Under the leadership of Stjepan Orešković, this program has contributed greatly to modern public health in other parts of the former Yugoslavia.

These leaders also have achieved much in the policy area, as illustrated by the effective programs against tobacco use in countries such as Poland and Croatia and also less visible work to promote reconciliation in the former Yugoslavia.

As these examples show, much has been achieved in Central and Eastern Europe, and more recently in the former Soviet Union, to prepare a new generation of leaders in health policy. Yet, there is still a great deal to be done. There are still many countries where public health capacity is almost nonexistent, with only a handful, if that, of individuals who understand the nature of the problem and what needs to be done. Inevitably, they are totally overstretched, as illustrated by the suggestion of one health minister that a particular individual should be able to develop a school of public health in the time left over from implementing a new health financing system. The problems are greatest in what was Soviet Central Asia and in those areas afflicted by war in the 1990s, such as the Caucasus and parts of Southeast Europe.

Lessons Learned

The picture painted in this chapter is largely one of success, but there have also been failures. A few schools of public health were launched to great acclaim but then withered. A significant number of those trained abroad either did not return to their home country or found employment in other areas, such as the pharmaceutical industry. As in Western countries, the impact of evidence on policy has often been less than desired. So what were the factors that determined whether there would be success or failure? In this section, I review briefly some of the issues involved.

Developing Career Opportunities

During the 1990s, many young people from former Communist countries received training in public health in the West. Many never returned. Yet, some countries were much more successful than others in retaining those who had been trained.

A key issue was whether the individual had something to return to that would provide a combination of financial security, opportunities for career progression, and intellectual stimulation. Too often, Western funding programs offered isolated scholarships with no thought about the individual's ultimate reentry to their country. Where overseas training was part of a larger reform program, as in Hungary, this was less of a problem because training went hand-in-hand with institutional development. Although on a smaller scale, this was also the case in the Russian program described. The Open Society Institute (Soros Foundation), which has made a major contribution to public health development in this region, provided reentry grants to support the integration of those returning and funding to strengthen their institutions. In contrast, where there was nothing to come back to or worse, where the home institutions remained unreformed, with elderly professors hostile to the threat posed by junior staff with ideas that contradicted everything they believed in, there was little reason to return.

Providing opportunities for those receiving training applies equally to those graduating from the new schools. The logical destination for many of their graduates would be the national public health systems. Unfortunately, there was often a mismatch between the obsolete ways these systems operated and the skills of the new graduates. The successful training programs had to engage actively with those working in public health to encourage change in the system and, in doing so, establish career pathways for their graduates. In the best examples, these recognized that master's level training is only the first step in a process of lifelong learning, strengthening the link further between academia and practice.

Securing Long-Term Funding

Public health knowledge is a public good in that once created, its use cannot be restricted to particular individuals, and one person's use of it does not reduce what is available for another. Public health infrastructure, including the institutions that generate and transmit this knowledge, is termed an access good, opening up opportunities to utilize the knowledge (Powles and Comim, 2003). As such, in a free market, public health infrastructure will attract inadequate investment.

In the early 1990s, when the international community's attention was still focused on the countries emerging from behind the Iron Curtain, funding from international development assistance, in particular the European Union and the World Bank, was available. However, it was always clear that such funding was only transitional; it was essential that the new schools of public health develop long-term, secure funding sources. The Communist model of fixed annual allocations to higher education institutions was gone; new arrangements involved competition for research and development funds, nationally and internationally, and the development of training courses of various types that responded to the needs of public health and other agencies and which they would pay for. The successful schools have achieved this, with the compact between the Hungarian school and the public health service an excellent example of an arrangement that brings benefits to both parties. For some, it has been more difficult. Thus, in the mid-1990s, institutions in, for example, Romania and the Czech Republic did not have accounting systems in place that would allow them to participate in European Union programs. This was still the case in many parts of the former Soviet Union in 2003. In some countries, this is exacerbated by factors such as poorly developed banking systems, making cash transfers difficult, and regulations on the import and export of money and equipment. And in many places, cash-strapped public health authorities simply do not have the funds available to pay for their staff to be trained. Consequently, there remains a considerable need for support by the international community of institutional development of schools of public health where they cannot yet hope to become economically viable on their own. However, this institutional support must go beyond training people in the technical aspects of public health: it must also encompass managerial, organizational, and fundraising skills.

Making a Difference

For public health to be valued, it must be seen as doing something useful. Public health leaders must contribute to national debates; problems that governments face in relation to public health are difficult, and they cannot expect to solve them on their own. Public health leaders, especially those in schools of public health, contribute to solving these problems. The most successful public health leaders have engaged in the policy process, with the greatest successes achieved by those working across government departments, in particular with finance ministries. Some of the best examples are from tobacco control, such as the work of Professor Witold Zatonski, who has contributed to Poland's having a tobacco policy much stricter than that in the European Union (Gilmore and Zatonski, 2002), or the campaign led by the Andrija Stampar School in Croatia (Marusic, 2002).

Effective public health leaders should not simply wait to be asked for their opinion. They should be advocates for health, drawing attention to issues that would otherwise be overlooked (Chapman, 2001). This requires a willingness to engage with the media, recognizing that journalists need stories; it is better if those stories promote rather than damage health. It also requires a proactive research agenda to understand the health challenges facing your population.

Yet, whereas advocacy is important, a cautionary note is necessary. Public health is based on social justice, so its advocates will often espouse causes that are unpopular, such as the rights of minorities—for example, the Roma population or drug users. In doing so, it is important not to become party political, recognizing the experience of Spain where, following the death of Franco, many of the new generation of public health professionals were closely allied with the Socialist Party and suffered when a right-wing government came to power in the 1990s.

Working Together Across Borders

The stories in this chapter represent the efforts of many people from different countries. The most successful have involved close cooperation between individuals and institutions in the East and the West, bringing mutual benefits. International cooperation has provided an opportunity to unlock much-needed funding sources but has gone beyond this, with shared research and collaborative training programs, such as the European Masters in Public Health, in which schools of public health from across Europe now collaborate (Cavallo, Rimpela, Normand, and Bury, 2001).

These collaborations have been possible only due to the availability of funding from various sources, in particular the European Union. However, they also owe much to the Europe-wide public health organizations that have striven to support the development of these newly emerging institutions. These are ASPHER, EUPHA, and the European Public Health Alliance (which brings together nongovernmental organizations). Each of these organizations has been helped greatly by the support of the Open Society Institute, which has worked with the European associations to develop twinning arrangements between organizations in the East and the West.

Conclusions

This brief account of experience in developing a new generation of public health leaders in the former Communist countries of Europe has been selective of necessity. There is much more that could be said. Nonetheless, certain lessons emerge.

The first is that the challenge faced has been different from that in many other parts of the world. The task was not to build something where nothing existed previously. Instead, it was to reorient a system that was already there but that was trapped in an ideological paradigm that, especially in the former Soviet Union, was incompatible with modern health. This called for particular skills, showing that change was needed but managing it in a way that was least threatening to those with the most to lose. The often-cited solution, retraining, has been of only moderate success, and regrettably, it has often been necessary to accept that some changes may take a generation to unfold.

The second is that there is still a substantial unfinished agenda in public health in this region. Much has been done but there is still much to do, and new threats are apparent, in particular from a combination of HIV and resistant tuberculosis and the predations of the global tobacco industry. Yet, this region remains a low priority on the international development agenda.

The third—and perhaps the most important—is the need for leadership. Where there has been success, there has been an individual who has displayed the features of effective leadership, who has become what Handy (1985) has described as a model for their team, inspiring their confidence, and an ambassador for them, advocating on their behalf and on behalf of the health of those of their compatriots. These individuals have possessed a clear vision: to create the opportunities to develop the new generation of public health professionals that their countries so need.

For others seeking to follow in their footsteps, several lessons emerge. By far the most important is the need to leave the classroom to engage with the wider world. A training program is of little value if it makes no attempt to identify and respond to the needs of those who will employ its graduates. An idea will come to fruition only if it can mobilize resources to sustain itself. This means engaging with governments and international agencies to change the agenda so that public health is seen as a priority. Most important, a school of public health will only be valued if it is seen to be contributing to society.

References

Andreev, E. M., McKee, M., and Shkolnikov, V. M. "Health Expectancy in Russia: A New Perspective on the Health Divide in Europe." *World Health Organization Bulletin*, forthcoming.

Andreev, E. M., and others. "The Evolving Pattern of Avoidable Mortality in Russia." *International Journal of Epidemiology*, 2003, *32*, 437–446.

Bojan, F., Belicza, E., Horvath, F., and McKee, M. "Teaching Public Health: An Innovative Method Using Computer-Based Project Work." *Medical Education*, 1995, *29*, 48–52.

Bojan, F., and McKee, M. "The Challenges to Public Health in Hungary in the 21st Century." *European Journal of Public Health*, 1997, *7*, 238–242.

Bojan, F., McKee, M., and Ostbye, T. "Status and Priorities of Public Health in Hungary." *Zeitschrift fur Gesundheitswissenschaften*, 1994, *Suppl. 1*, 48–55.

Borovecki, A., Belicza, B., and Orešković, S. "75th Anniversary of Andrija Stampar School of Public Health—What Can We Learn from Our Past for the Future?" *Croatian Medical Journal*, 2002, *43*, 371–373.

Bosma, H., and others. "Differences in Mortality and Coronary Heart Disease Between Lithuania and The Netherlands: Results from the WHO Kaunas-Rotterdam Intervention Study (KRIS)." *International Journal of Epidemiology*, 1994, *23*, 12–19.

Cavallo, F., Rimpela, A., Normand, C., and Bury, J. "Public Health Training in Europe: Development of European Masters Degrees in Public Health." *European Journal of Public Health*, 2001, *11*, 171–173.

Chapman, S. "Advocacy in Public Health: Roles and Challenges." *International Journal of Epidemiology*, 2001, *30*, 1226–1232.

Chenet, L., and others. "Changing Life Expectancy in Central Europe: Is There a Single Reason?" *Journal of Public Health Medicine*, 1996, *18*, 329–336.

Dolea, C., Nolte, E., and McKee, M. "Changing Life Expectancy in Romania After the Transition." *Journal of Epidemiology and Community Health*, 2002, *56*, 444–449.

Field, M. G. "Noble Purpose, Grand Design, Flawed Execution, Mixed Results: Soviet Socialized Medicine After Seventy Years." *American Journal of Public Health*, 1990, *80*, 144–145.

Gilmore, A., and Zatonski, W. "Free Trade v. the Protection of Health: How Will EU Accession Influence Tobacco Control in Poland?" *Eurohealth*, 2002, *8*(4), 31–33.

Gjonca, A. *Communism, Health, and Lifestyle: The Paradox of Mortality Transition in Albania, 1950–1990*. Westport, Conn.: Greenwood Press, 2001.

Gribbin, J. *Science: A History*. London: Penguin Books, 2003.

Hamers, F. F., and Downs, A. M. "HIV in Central and Eastern Europe." *Lancet*, 2003, *361*, 1035–1044.

Handy, C. B. *Understanding Organizations*. London: Penguin Books, 1985.

Healy, J., and McKee, M. "Implementing Hospital Reform in Central and Eastern Europe." *Health Policy*, 2002, *61*, 1–19.

Joravsky, D. *The Lysenko Affair*. Chicago: University of Chicago Press, 1970.

Kalediene, R. "Resources for Development of Training in Public Health and Health Management in Eastern Europe: The Kaunas Experience." *Public Health Review*, 2002, *30*, 145–154.

Kohler, L., and Eklund L. "BRIMHEALTH: A Successful Experience in Nordic-Baltic Co-operation in Public Health Training." *European Journal of Public Health*, 2002, *12*, 152–154.

Kozinetz, C., Matusa, R., and Cazazu, A. "The Changing Epidemic of Pediatric HIV Infection in Romania." *Annals of Epidemiology*, 2000, *10*, 474–475.

Krementsov, N. L. *Stalinist Science*. Princeton, N.J.: Princeton University Press, 1997.

Marusic, A. "Croatia Opens a National Centre for the Prevention of Smoking." *Lancet*, 2002, *359*, 954.

McKee, M. "The Health Effects of the Collapse of the Soviet Union." In
    D. Leon and G. Walt (eds.), *Poverty, Inequality and Health*. Oxford,
    U.K.: Oxford University Press, 2001, pp. 17–36.

McKee, M., Bojan, F., White, M., and Ostbye, T. "Development of Public Health
    Training in Hungary—An Exercise in International Co-operation." *Journal
    of Public Health Medicine*, 1995, *17*, 438–444.

McKee, M., and others. "Health Policy-Making in Central and Eastern Europe:
    Lessons from the Inaction on Injuries?" *Health Policy Planning*, 2000, *15*,
    263–269.

McMichael, A. J., McKee, M., Shkolnikov, V., and Valkonen, T. "Mortality
    Trends and Setbacks: Global Convergence or Divergence?" *Lancet*, 2002,
    363, 1155–1159.

Powles, J., and Comim, F. "Public Health Infrastructure and Knowledge." In
    R. Smith, R. Beaglehole, D. Woodward, and N. Drager (eds.), *Global
    Public Goods for Health*. Oxford, U.K.: Oxford University Press, 2003,
    pp. 159–173.

Soyfer, V. N. "The Consequences of Political Dictatorship for Russian Science."
    Nature Review of Genetics, 2001, *2*, 723–729.

Tkatchenko, E., McKee, M., and Tsouros, A. D. "Public Health in Russia:
    The View from the Inside." *Health Policy Planning*, 2000, *15*, 164–169.

Tokin, B. P., and others. *o Biologii*. Moscow: Partizdat, 1936.

Tunstall-Pedoe, H., and others. "Contribution of Trends in Survival and
    Coronary-Event Rates to Changes in Coronary Heart Disease Mortality:
    10-Year Results from 37 WHO MONICA Project Populations. Monitor-
    ing Trends and Determinants in Cardiovascular Disease." *Lancet*, 1999,
    353, 1547–1557.

Walberg P., and others. "Economic Change, Crime, and Mortality Crisis in Rus-
    sia: A Regional Analysis." *BMJ*, 1998, *317*, 312–318.

White, M., Watt, I., Bojan, F., and McKee, M. "Hungary: A New Public Health."
    Lancet, 1993, *341*, 43–44.

Zatonski, W. A., McMichael, A. J., and Powles, J. W. "Ecological Study of Rea-
    sons for Sharp Decline in Mortality from Ischaemic Heart Disease in
    Poland Since 1991." *BMJ*, 1998, *316*, 1047–1051.

14

Building the Next
Generation of Leaders

Joy Phumaphi

Global health is a public good in a dynamic, expanding, and increasingly complex market and even more demanding clientele. Today has, more than ever before, become the end of yesterday and the beginning of tomorrow. The health challenges of today require building on lessons learned from past successes and failures of everyone. Attaining the targets set by the global community requires a new type of leader: one who will follow, support, develop skills, and still come out in front.

A Needs Assessment

Today's leader not only must have leadership potential but also must be a product of comprehensive education in a dynamic environment. The people we serve will only get the required response from a leader if the leader understands the needs of the community he or she serves.

In the past century, a new era in global health has evolved and matured. Evidence-based interventions were developed for addressing the majority of health challenges contributing to the bulk of the global disease burden. The following examples of tools that were identified and that have progressively become more accessible illustrate this point:

- An increased number of vaccines between 1923 and 1992, including among others diphtheria, pertussis, tuberculosis, tetanus, yellow fever, polio, measles, mumps, rubella, hepatitis, and *Haemophilus influenzae* type B

- The fluoridation of water (a great public health triumph available to all)

- Effective management programs for chronic illnesses such as diabetes and high blood pressure and the prevention of the same life-threatening conditions and killer diseases such as cancers

- Effective interventions and tools for reproductive health, as well as the management of childhood illnesses that, when applied, could lead to a surpassing of the Millennium Development Goals

This was accompanied by the introduction of primary health care systems that established essential pillars such as health promotion, which has become one of the greatest contributions to sustainable health care. Essential care can now be based on practical, scientifically sound, and socially acceptable methods and technology. Health care has been made universally accessible to individuals and families in the community through their full participation and at a cost that the community and country can afford to maintain at every stage of their development through self-reliance and self-determination.

Many communities have developed strong areas in their health systems and service delivery over the years. Several weaknesses still need to be addressed, opportunities taken advantage of, and challenges met.

Health leaders must understand this environment and appreciate that the circle of concern in the health sector extends beyond the public and private sectors. They have an equal responsibility to understand the work of the volunteer movements, nongovernmental organizations (NGOs), community-based organizations, and the traditional sector. Understanding, however, is not enough; linkages have to be forged not only with these groups but also with other sectors that support the health sector—planning, finance, agriculture, trade, utilities (water, energy), and communication—to best respond to community needs, withstand change, and ensure sustainability.

Opportunities for collaboration and partnerships are constantly presenting themselves at every level. Development initiatives, whether internally or externally funded, present possibilities for health. The building of a road means being able to work with transporters to offer transportation to mothers to be able to access perinatal care or children for routine immunizations in remote areas. The construction of a school offers access to households through their children to carry out health promotion. Even with new challenges to global health, such as HIV/AIDS (human immunodeficiency virus–acquired immunodeficiency syndrome) and severe acute respiratory syndrome (SARS), there is greater understanding of the system barriers that impede progress and the implementation of the necessary interventions. The best predictor of the future is the past, and leaders who thoroughly understand this will have the capacity to both create and catch a new vision.

To overcome the challenges facing these areas, public health leaders at international, national, state, local, and community levels need to be familiar with these challenges to become advocates and to garner increased commitment to obtaining adequate resources for equipment, supplies, infrastructure, human resources, support systems, and running expenses.

Global Challenges: Local Context

The diversity of the determinants of health, combined with the potential effects of varying global trends and events, makes it absolutely critical for the current generation of leaders to know as much as possible about applying global market characteristics and expectations to local environments.

Income and social status can be the biggest and most difficult barriers to access to adequate health care. Social support networks that exist in different communities can be valuable partners, persistent irritants, or looming threats, depending on how they are engaged. The level of education and literacy in a community determines to a large extent the responsiveness of families and individuals to health promotion and their use of health services. Employment and working conditions, social environments, physical environments, geography, politics, personal health practices and coping skills, development programs, biology and genetic endowment, the nature of health services, gender, and culture all need to be understood in the local context. Failure to recognize and pay respect to a traditional leader in many African communities has resulted in the failure of many development efforts.

It is critical, therefore, that in aligning global goals to local expectations, the interventions required be made country-specific; in addition, indicators that are developed should be country-specific rather than global averages. Before accepting plans, leaders must ascertain that district priorities have been appraised and that targets and objectives for health care respond to local needs. District action plans for important programs must form the basis for national programs. This makes it easier to identify the key players, their agenda, and effects on the local environment so that effective partnerships can be developed and their ideal roles and relationships defined in the domestic, regional, and global arenas.

Framework: Using a Mix of Partners

A leader who tries to drive the health agenda alone lacks vision. A vision from the creative stages must be transmitted, much like a virus, to everyone. Setting the goals for a national strategy then becomes a positive experience for everyone. Every stakeholder needs to feel a part of the solution. To reach this point, all must see the problem. There is an old African proverb about some blind men who were asked to describe an elephant. One got hold of its trunk and said that the elephant was like a long, thick snake. Another felt the leg and said it resembled a tree trunk. The next ran his palm along its broad side and said it was like a wall. The fourth touched its hard, sharp tusk and likened the elephant to a horn. The last carefully caressed the big ears and was convinced that the elephant was similar to a fan.

It is difficult for everyone to see the same vision or to interpret a challenge in the same way because we all experience life differently. There must therefore be effective mechanisms for getting everyone on board. This is particularly important because not only are the players diverse, but the challenge itself is complex.

Life expectancy varies among economic groupings, in communities, in countries, and among countries. The average in the industrialized countries is seventy-three years compared with fifty years in Africa. The same can be said for infant mortality, which varies between nine per one thousand in the industrialized countries and an average of ninety-seven per one thousand in Africa.

The gaps in global health are many and varied. In 2003, the World Health Organization (WHO) and UNAIDS declared the gap in antiretroviral treatment of HIV/AIDS patients a global emergency. Leaders cannot lose sight of this or the responsibility to plug these gaps, such as the "10/90 gap" wherein less than 10 percent of the worldwide expenditure on health research and development is devoted to the major health problems of 90 percent of the global population.

Research that could inform behavioral change interventions is lagging far behind in the war against HIV/AIDS; yet, this is the area where the spread of the deadly virus could be interrupted. It would address issues such as intergenerational sex and turning the tide of the rapid transmission among young people.

Health leaders must ensure that an action plan reinforces the weak areas by taking advantage of opportunities and building on and using strengths.

National priorities must be set with the full understanding of the needs of the population and the implications of every choice. Once the resources are available, there also must be adequate incentives, logistics, and organizational arrangements to ensure the prompt delivery of services. This is the responsibility of every global leader, just as much as it is the responsibility of every head of state and minister of finance and health to ensure that health expenditure as a percentage of the gross domestic product (GDP) indicates the priority of health on the country's development agenda. Per capita income spent on health in the United States is 13 percent, or U.S.$4,093, whereas in most African countries it is between 2 and 3 percent, or between U.S.$1 and U.S.$5.

Leadership in health is not the preserve of national actors but extends to global partnerships with other governments, agencies, international organizations, and corporations. Understanding the environment in which programs are introduced is a critical leadership responsibility for these partners.

The poor understanding of this complex relationship led to the devastation wreaked on the health sector by the structural adjustment programs of the 1980s. Restrictions on borrowing and government expenditure led to the cutting of critical pillars in primary heath care delivery. Wage cuts and price increases in communities where a single breadwinner supports a large extended family led to poor nutrition, limited access to education and health services, and a collapse of a social support structure that was the mainstay of rural and periurban development. This misguided management of limited resources only increased the debt burden and led to a vicious circle of reduced health expenditure, user fees (cost recovery), limited access, poor health, reduced opportunities for education, unemployment, and poverty.

The effects on maternal mortality and morbidity of structural adjustment program–user charges for antenatal and maternity care have been associated with increases in deliveries at home (without skilled attendants), rising costs of transportation, and denied emergency obstetrical care.

The effect of structural adjustment programs on child nutrition has been well documented by the United Nations Coordinating Committee subcommittee on nutrition when reporting on the deterioration in child nutritional status in sub-Saharan Africa between 1975 and 1990 (United Nations, 1992). In many countries, this contributed to higher infant and child mortality and morbidity. The structural adjustment programs led to declines in income and increases in food prices combined with health expenditure cutbacks in preventative programs, resulting in the deterioration in both quantity and quality of diets, immunizations coverage, utilization of health services for acute conditions, and the weakening of disease control programs. The abrupt denial of access to health care services in some communities led to the revival of home remedies at a time when people who had the knowledge had stopped passing it on. In some areas, this set health care back decades.

Working together, global and local leaders in health can respond to local needs in an effective and sustainable manner. Integrated primary health care systems are not just the usual choice, they are the logical choice. The health challenge is difficult enough without partners frustrating each other's efforts. A good leader has happy colleagues in the public, private, traditional, and NGO sectors.

Successful integration leads to increased job satisfaction among health care workers, improved patient service, improved community health, and less inefficient use of the health care system. One of the most telling tragedies of the HIV/AIDS epidemic for health professionals has been the loss of confidence, demoralization, and inefficiency caused by having to see most of their patients die without responding to treatment for opportunistic infections. The "3-by-5 initiative" (a global call to action to distribute anti-retroviral therapy to three million people in fifty developing countries by the end of 2005) will change the face of health service in the affected countries in more ways than one.

Good community integration ensures the following features:

- Focuses on the individual

- Starts with primary health

- Shares information and exploits technology

- Creates virtual networks at various levels

- Develops needs-based funding models

- Implements a mechanism for monitoring and evaluation

Guiding the development, implementation, and monitoring of the action plan must be based on integration at the functional, health professional, and clinical levels.

Some practical advice would be:

- Start with the individual and the family. Never forget that you need to be healthy to contribute toward development.

- Use primary health care because it entails partnership with the community and the development of a strong prevention pillar that can never be replaced by any other approach.

- Allow the stakeholders to share information vertically and horizontally and exploit technology because primary health care is *not* second-rate care!

- Create networks at all levels, both physically in the community and on the Internet (virtual networks).

- Study financing models and select one that will not deny people access to health care. If necessary, develop a special model.

- Build management, monitoring, and evaluation mechanisms into the plan and ensure that it has a time frame with milestones and indicators.

The lack of regular monitoring with quality assurance and evaluation tools continues to be the major cause of the collapse of health programs and systems.

Leaders who leave stakeholders out must make sure that they are not needed or that they cannot sabotage the plan. If this rule is applied, leaders have to work with everyone. By engaging the individual, the family, and the community, the changes that give more power to these important health partners is fully supported and reinforced by the health professionals.

Implementing the Strategy—Using a People-Centered Approach

Health care is a basic human right that must be available and accessible in a sustainable manner to all at all times. Human resources are not only pivotal and critical to health services delivery, they are a health leader's most valuable ally. Although infrastructure development requirements are key, facilities have to be staffed by trained professionals. Although drugs and technology are often taken to constitute the most essential element of care and treatment, they need trained professionals for them to be used safely and efficaciously. Financial resources have to be managed by human resources in order for them to purchase the required service. Every single resource needs human capital for it to play its role.

A new leader puts people at the center in an approach to health care that emphasizes preventive, promotive, and curative services. The efficient, effective, and economic delivery of this service entails good governance, which is as critical to health service delivery as it is to any other sector. Prompt, equitable, and professional services must become a cardinal principle for all, starting with the leader.

Putting people first means empowering them at a grassroots level to be responsible health partners. It also means strengthening clinics, health centers, hospitals, and support services to address the primary health challenges such as child survival, adolescent health services, maternal survival, noncommunicable diseases, mental health, emergencies and injuries, and male involvement. This entails providing motivation and incentives for the players in the health system and clearly defining their administrative and participatory roles, with limits and jurisdictions. It means decentralizing powers, training all participants, and broadening the operational base.

To do this, leaders must appreciate that the relationship between economics and health is one of the oldest social relationships in our societies. Some of the first currency in rudimentary trade (barter) was food. This was critical to the health status of people. Over the years, the relationship has remained definite but increasingly more complex. One common complicating factor is that per capita income alone will not improve health status, but income distribution must be such that everyone earns enough to satisfy basic human needs of shelter, clothing, access to health services, education, water, and choices for self-actualization. Many health economists believe that the disease burden and patterns experienced by the developing countries are strikingly similar to those of nineteenth-century Europe. They are primarily diseases of underdevelopment and poverty, not a feature of warm climates in the tropics. Full integration with development planning and other sectors, the involvement of all stakeholders, and building partnerships is a continuous process that must be constantly nurtured.

Managing resources and ensuring sustainability are about thinking outside the box and exploring new territory. There is no magic bullet. There are, however, certain prerequisites that, if safeguarded, can inject some magic into the service.

Protecting standards and quality, enhancing performance, using operational research—these are steps that move the interventions upstream and save considerably more money for the economy as a whole while leaving people healthier.

Enter the Global Leaders

The thrill of the challenge is often brought into sharper focus by a global perspective, which necessarily requires leaders to understand visions, targets, and missions of other leaders playing under different rules. Shifting from a local to a global perspective increases the complexity of the challenge and opens leaders to the effects of globalization.

Learning global culture entails first of all understanding the economic importance of effective health care. From the point of view of individual health providers, it is easiest to see illnesses as isolated episodes. However, from a household and national point of view, the welfare of the breadwinner (and dependents), caregiver, and student is critical to income levels, expenditure levels, development of future potential, and overall socioeconomic well-being. From this perspective, national health makes both practical and economic sense.

The tremendous cost of ill health is reflected in the quality of life, loss of working hours, poor-quality work, and reduced potential. Experience has clearly demonstrated that it is far more expensive to treat illness than to prevent it in the first place. Movement of people, trade, natural disasters, security, development agendas, and international as well as bilateral agreements influence health outcomes.

Global leaders must see this big picture, embracing change and technology while internalizing the past. Countries that are far behind have an opportunity to skip a step or two and move higher up the technology ladder without having to worry about a commitment to existing infrastructure. The use of consumer-centered information and even telemedicine then becomes only logical. The Iran government recently made a decision to follow this route following the Ban earthquake.

A performance-oriented culture has not detracted from the fact that leaders shall always need the ability to hold court: to consult in a manner that ensures ownership without compromising on guidance.

Essential qualities of a good leader continue to apply because he or she requires—in addition to basic knowledge—drive, initiative, sensitivity, passion, attitude, value system, and a mental toughness that guarantees staying power. Possessing unlimited energy, global thinkers must be problem solvers who can synthesize; are innovative and intuitive; and have heightened senses, tenacity, good negotiating skills, resilience, and the ability to do many things at once.

Accepting their own weaknesses, leaders must respect the traits of others. Whereas many health providers take the view that their profession is an end in itself to health care delivery, it is clear that health care systems can only be successful at providing health care if they are integrated into the larger economic fabric of life.

Conclusion

Every health leader has to be driven by the "Health for All" vision. It is the attainment by all citizens of the globe by 2000 of a level of health that would permit them to lead socially and economically productive lives. It is a holistic view of health defined within the socioeconomic construct of a rapidly developing world. It is based on the principles of equity and solidarity, which emphasize individual, family, and community responsibility for health within the overall development framework of a society. Today's global leaders must protect this noble goal. The year 2000 is long past, but the vision must live on within a constructive spirit of discontent that is critical enough to remove the barriers that are hindering this global agenda.

We all must be willing to take responsibility and share the joy of accomplishment. Only then can the true potential energies of this global force work successfully for the benefit of mankind.

Disclaimer: The views expressed in this contribution are those of the writer and do not necessarily reflect the position, decisions, or stated policy of any organization or group with whom the writer is associated.

Reference

United Nations. *Second Report on the World Nutrition Situation*. Vols. I and II. Geneva: United Nations, 1992.

15

Creating Public Health Leaders

Public Health Leadership Institutes

William L. Roper and Janet Porter

Health ministries, governmental agencies, and foundations have been investing in relief and health infrastructure programs for developing nations for decades. Public health issues in developing nations are complex, and interventions are challenging to execute successfully. Thus, programmatic interventions and understanding of the implementation of these programs have met with mixed results. The realities of political instability, poverty, and war in many developing nations result in suboptimal investment and use of existing resources and knowledge that produce less constructive outcomes. Process and outcomes are not widely evaluated in developing countries, and as a result, limited problem-solving knowledge is generated. All of these factors have been found to be hampered by the lack of in-country leadership and managerial skills to support design and execution of programmatic interventions.

Clearly, a constraining factor in the improvement of health status in many developing nations is the lack of leadership and management skills. Health systems cannot be run effectively unless leaders and managers are skilled in assessment, planning, budgeting,

The authors would like to thank Sue Zelt, M.P.H., M.B.A., a doctoral student in the department of health policy and administration, University of North Carolina–Chapel Hill School of Public Health, for her contributions to this chapter.

program development, and oversight. Leadership skills are required to translate policy into implementable projects and programs to ensure the availability of human and financial resources. Many public health managers in developing countries also generally lack the understanding of the organizational and systemic contexts within which they operate. Globally, leadership is critically needed to identify and promote cost-effective approaches to health and facilitate the activities of public and nongovernmental providers.

Importance of Leadership Development in Developing Nations

Although difficult to assess, investments in improved health status in 2003 were at best stagnant and likely to decline in the future. However, the number of agencies supporting health programs appears to be increasing, and coordinating these efforts has become more complex (Walt, Pavignani, Gilson, and Buse, 1999). A response to sustaining this growing health care sector in developing nations with less aid is a call for better management and leadership. Therefore, leadership development is considered crucial to maintaining the health sector.

Likewise, powerful foundations, such as the Bill and Melinda Gates Foundation, that demand measurable outcomes are creating a new global aid paradigm. More than ever before, the expectation is for a demonstrated return of investment to ensure continued funding.

Evaluation studies conducted by the World Health Organization (WHO) and other agencies have shown that interventions in developing countries have been limited in their effectiveness by the inability of ministries of health to effectively develop and execute strategies and systems for the consistent delivery of drugs, health equipment, and other services to those in need. Some of the causes of these impediments are the lack of established policies and procedures and inherent management system deficiencies in logistics, information systems, client referral and tracking, supervision, evaluations, and monitoring of interventions. Moreover, studies have consistently demonstrated that political leaders in developing nations use aid programs for their own political advantage without regard to the health and welfare of their own people.

These evaluations clearly illustrate the need to build and support leadership capacity in developing nations. The development of leadership skills in developing countries should be focused on policy formulation and programmatic implementation, monitoring, and evaluation, particularly for key stakeholders in ministries of health and nongovernmental organizations (NGOs). Building leadership capacity and critical mass through the understanding and development of infrastructure such as logistics, information systems, client registration, supervision, and monitoring systems is also critical.

Public Health Leadership Development in the United States

The 1988 Institute of Medicine (IOM) report, *The Future of Public Health*, was a clarion call domestically for an investment in leadership development among public health professionals. This report identified that the vast majority of the senior leaders in public health had no formal management or leadership training, having earned medical degrees or degrees in public health or nursing. Furthermore, the field of public health did not have consensus about the importance of scholarship around public health leadership. A mere eight years later, another IOM (1996) report, *Healthy Communities: New Partnerships for the Future of Public Health*, concluded that progress has been made in public health leadership development in the United States. It is interesting to note that progress has been made through nondegree programs targeted at midcareer public health professionals. Little change has occurred in terms of degree-granting education for those entering the field of public health professionals. For example, the Commission on Education for

Public Health, the accrediting body for schools and programs in public health, has not developed standards related to the leadership curriculum of master's degree programs in public health. Nor have master's or doctoral programs in public health leadership been developed. Thus, the progress that has been made has been with midcareer and senior careerists rather than early careerists.

Much of the credit goes to the Centers for Disease Control and Prevention (CDC), which made the primary investment, beginning with the establishment of the National Public Health Leadership Institute (PHLI) in 1991. At the same time, state and regional public health leadership developments began to be established, with seed money coming from CDC, supplemented by contracts with state governments and foundation support. Today, sixteen state and regional public health leadership institutes, along with PHLI, belong to the National Leadership Network, a consortium focused on strengthening the scholarship about public health leadership and the sharing of best practices among programs.

The state, regional, and national programs have similar objectives but vary in curricula, format, length, admission process, and participant expectations. To understand the variation in programs all designed to strengthen public health leadership skills, we will describe a few of the programs. The PHLI, sponsored by CDC, is currently administered by a partnership between the School of Public Health and the Kenan-Flagler Business School of the University of North Carolina at Chapel Hill and the Center for Creative Leadership. Teams of fifty-five senior leaders in public health from both the public and private sectors attend the yearlong programs. The program is designed to challenge senior leaders to reflect on their own leadership characteristics, to develop leadership skills, and to apply their leadership skills to a personally selected leadership challenge. The philosophy is that skills are honed through practice; the leadership teams are expected to practice their newly acquired skills on the project they must complete and present within the PHLI year. Since its inception, more than seven hundred senior public health leaders have completed PHLI.

The legacy of the program lies not only in the cadre of public health leaders who attribute their leadership skills and current leadership positions to PHLI but also in the Public Health Leadership Society, the national alumni organization that promotes lifelong leadership learning and networking. Impact evaluations have consistently shown that PHLI has a transformational effect on many of the PHLI scholars. PHLI is distinguished from the state and regional leadership institutes in that scholars are drawn from a national—and even international—audience, they are in more senior positions, and they are in leadership positions in both public and private settings.

Typical of the sixteen state and regional public health leadership programs, the Southeast Public Health Leadership Institute is a yearlong leadership development program for state and local government public health leaders in five states: Virginia, South Carolina, North Carolina, Tennessee, and West Virginia. Supported primarily by state contracts, the forty midlevel public health leaders apply and attend as individuals. The content has traditionally been similar to that of PHLI, with a focus on transformational leadership skills: negotiating, partnerships, risk communication, and visioning. The infusion of bioterrorism funding following the attacks of September 11, 2001, has resulted in a change in both the background of applicants and program content with a theme of crisis management.

A newer program, funded in response to the dearth of minorities in senior leadership positions in public health, is the Emerging Leaders in Public Health program, funded by the W. K. Kellogg Program. The interest—and availability—of midlevel and senior minorities in public health was evident when the program, designed exclusively for minorities, had more than 175 applicants for the first cohort of 32. With about one-third of the first cohort African Americans, one-third American Indians, and one-third Hispanics, this program applies general leadership theories to some of the unique challenges faced by minorities in leadership roles. Like the previously mentioned programs, this yearlong program selects currently employed public health professionals and enrolls them in a program with some residential (face-to-face) education, extensive distance learning (teleconferences, Internet discussion groups, simulations), 360-degree personal leadership development and coaching, and the expectations of practicing leadership skills through a personal leadership project.

What do these domestic public health leadership programs have in common? First, they have as a foundation the knowledge gained from years of leadership research across government and private industry, foundations, and community organizations. As one notable example, the thirty-year-old nonprofit International Center for Creative Leadership development programs, ranked number 1 by *Business Week* in leadership development ("Exec-Ed Rankings and Profiles," 2003), conducts research, develops new products and services to strengthen leadership skills, offers leadership development programs using those products and services, and then conducts extensive research on the efficacy of those services. The center's research consistently has found that skills deficits and leadership development needs are similar across all industries and sectors. Therefore, like master's programs in business administration whose premise is that management skills are generic and applicable across all industries, most of the Center for Creative Leadership's programs and products are applicable to leaders regardless of age, sex, ethnicity, race, or professional training. The domestic public health leadership programs are committed to integrating the most contemporary thinking about leadership development from organizations like the Center for Creative Leadership and business and public administration faculty in notable institutions.

Second, the programs are designed with an appreciation of how adults learn. Edgar Dale's (1969) forty years of research has demonstrated that adults learn by reflection, application, and active engagement. So all the leadership programs minimize lecture, using instead case studies, exercises, role playing, and simulations to engage the leaders in their own development. The action-learning format continues with the expectation that participants apply their new skills to public health projects that interest them and are a priority to the communities they serve. In this way, participants are both learning by practicing new skills and also affecting the health status in their communities.

Third, all the programs use both residential and distance learning to create professional learning communities. Discussion forums, teleconferences, videoconferences, and Internet-based courses are used to connect the public health leaders with each other and to maximize peer learning. Software programs are becoming more facile in engaging and networking the participants so that they stick with the learning process despite the pressing challenges of their positions.

Fourth, the programs recognize that leadership skills acquisition and modifying behavior take a long time. Leadership skills are not developed by attending a two-day continuing education workshop. Rather, an intensive, long commitment to personal leadership development with support from faculty and coaches is required to have sustained improvement in leadership effectiveness.

Finally, the programs recognize that leadership development programs vary along a pedagogical continuum in terms of the emphasis placed on "reflection" versus "action" learning. Arguably, there are two schools of thought about the way leaders should be developed. Proponents of the reflection model argue that leaders learn through personal self-awareness and reflection; proponents of the action model believe that leaders learn through action—challenging new assignments, failure, mentoring and coaching others, and the like. To differentiate the two models, reflection programs place greater emphasis on

- 360-degree assessment instruments: colleagues, supervisors, subordinates, and customers provide feedback to the individual about their strengths and weaknesses.

- Personalized coaching and the development of a personal leadership development plan that addresses strengthening individual weaknesses.

- Storytelling: the leaders are expected to reflect on and then verbalize their own leadership histories, their leadership concepts, and their relationships with mentors and role models.

- Journaling: leaders are expected to reflect in writing in a private diary the lessons learned and develop plans to apply those lessons to their current position.

Action leadership development programs emphasize

- Cases, simulations, debates, role playing, games, and so on to actively engage participants in skill building

- Challenging assignments—such as switching jobs for six months with a peer—to stretch an individual's perspective and rapidly acquire skills

- Field trips to benchmarked organizations—firms the leadership aspires to emulate—to see improved performance in action

- Projects that challenge the leaders to apply their skills acquisition to relevant challenges from their organizations

Recognizing that individual learning styles vary, programs employ both the reflection and the action approach, with some programs placing greater emphasis on reflection and others placing greater emphasis on action.

Interestingly, the need for leadership development programs in developing countries was identified as a key issue before the recognition of the need in the United States. However, the relatively rapid development, endorsement, and success of public health leadership development programs has not been capitalized on by those interested in leadership programs in developing countries. A key question to ask is, "What can the leadership programs from developing countries learn from the domestic experience—and what can the U.S. programs learn from the better-established international programs?"

Leadership Development Programs for Developing Countries

Public health leadership development programs vary greatly throughout the world. The formats of programs include Web-based learning, teleconferencing, and face-to-face seminars. The length of commitment to leadership development by international public health professionals can vary from weeks to as long as six years. The process of leadership development may include a series of internships at public health agencies, formalized curriculum, or a combination of both practices. The following are brief descriptions of some of the various types of leadership development programs for developing nations.

Leadership development programming is supported through formalized fellowships, such as the yearlong Hubert H. Humphrey Fellowship program and the Fogarty Fellowship for the development of a cadre of young foreign investigators who work with U.S. scientists to understand disease pathogenesis, anticipate disease trends, and develop interventions. Both of these competitive programs select leaders from around the world—for example, in the case of the Humphrey program, for 2003–2004, 140 leaders were selected from more than 3,000 applicants. Similarly, the Population Fellows Programs, funded by the U.S. Agency for International Development (USAID) and other donors and administered by the University of Michigan School of Public Health, Ann Arbor, is designed to further the professional development of those building careers in international family planning and reproductive health over a two-year commitment. USAID also funds the Public Health Institute's Population Leadership Program, which is targeted for midlevel and senior-level international public health professionals. These highly trained leaders use their skills developed through these fellowships to make changes in their respective countries' health care systems. All of these programs are focused on action learning, skills development, and knowledge acquisition with the participants actively engaged in classes, assignments, and the like. Less emphasis is placed on individual leadership skills assessments, reflection, and coaching.

International public health programs leading to master's degrees in public health are also offered by many public health schools in the United States. Most notable are programs at the Johns Hopkins University in Baltimore, Maryland, and the Harvard School of Public Health in Cambridge, Massachusetts. Harvard University also offers a nondegree managing health program in developing countries involving two-month intensive workshops designed for the development of midlevel health care professionals. Many of the students in international public health programs are from developing nations and return to their native countries to use their formal education to improve the health in their country.

The CDC's Sustainable Management Development Program is a six-week intensive residential program designed to improve the effectiveness of public health programs by strengthening management-training capability in developing countries. The intensive residential program is followed by in-country consultation. The "train-the-trainer" program builds capacity by strengthening the teaching knowledge and skills of faculty in developing nations. Ultimately, the CDC aims to build a global network of sustainable management development programs that provide skills and competencies to public health managers throughout the developing world.

The World Bank Early Childhood Development (ECD) Virtual University targets ECD professionals through a predominantly distance-learning environment to encourage partnerships and capacity building among institutes, governments, employers, NGOs, students, and teachers to ultimately strengthen regional capacity to plan, implement, and evaluate ECD programs. The ECD Virtual University enrolls thirty committed professionals from across Africa who ultimately facilitate the interaction of ECD country-based networks with the ideas shared and generated through the program.

The Bill and Melinda Gates Institute for Population and Reproductive Health provides strategic leadership training seminars in Asia, Africa, and Latin America and develops interactive leadership training materials to support effective family planning, reproductive health, and population programs. To date, this program has trained more than four hundred reproductive health leaders from Africa, Asia, and Latin America.

Project Hope is a partnership with Johnson & Johnson, Inc., to increase the management skills of midlevel health care managers in the Czech Republic and Hungary. The four-week program is designed to improve the effectiveness and efficiency of health care facilities through better management, to increase coordination and networking among participants, and to encourage teamwork and combine theory and practice. The program is based on team training and addresses the following core themes: the role of management, strategy and implementation, operations management and quality improvement, human resources, finance and budgeting, and project planning. Sixty managers in three-member teams are selected from hospitals each year. Participants are invited to report the status of the project implementation on a yearly basis. Through the course, participants develop a regional network of colleagues for support in their work.

IntraHealth International is an affiliate of the University of North Carolina at Chapel Hill whose mission is to improve the quality and accessibility of health care services for people in need around the globe. Their focus is on improving the performance of health care providers and health service organizations; strengthening the work and service-policy environments of health care workers; developing responsive training and learning solutions for health services; and integrating nontraining solutions, including supervision, provider, motivation, and process improvement. The current programs implemented by IntraHealth are primarily funded by USAID. Whereas IntraHealth International's target audience is more entry-level, Management Sciences for Health (MSH) focuses more on senior leaders in public health.

Lead International offers an eighteen-month international training program in leadership for sustainable development. This fellowship is designed to focus participants on learning by doing through international and regional assignments and workshops. The main focus of the Lead International fellowship is to build a network of professionals to strengthen cross-cultural communication, problem solving, and decision making and to build effective analytical and presentation skills. For the past decade, Lead International has offered a unique eighteen-month international training program in leadership for sustainable development. "Lead Fellows"—graduates of the program—currently number about twelve hundred in seventy countries. They belong to the worlds of academia, business, government, media, and NGOs.

Winrock International is a global nonprofit organization headquartered in Morrilton, Arkansas, that works with others to increase economic opportunity, sustain natural resources, and protect the environment. Winrock offers nondegree Web-based programs that are designed to engage women, girls, and their male allies in lifetime commitments to social justice causes and economic advancement. Ultimately, Winrock International seeks to develop a network of activists to bring about changes in policies, programs, and practices that affect people in poverty. For the past four decades, Winrock International has been setting standards for programs to identify and develop potential leaders. An example of the solutions that Winrock International's leadership development programs produce are the African Women Leaders in Agriculture and the Environment program, which has reached thousands of women in ten countries. The program empowers women to enter new fields and change the course of institutions and agencies in rural areas in developing nations.

These programs offer a variety of approaches to strengthening leadership of public health professionals in developing nations. USAID and other key funding agencies have recognized the need for leadership development as a first infrastructure element that precedes the arrival of other aid.

Conclusion

Clearly there is a need for in-country leadership and managerial skills to support the design and execution of programmatic intervention in developing nations. Leadership skills are required to identify and promote cost-effective approaches to health and facilitate public health activities. Numerous organizations and programs have addressed this need for leadership development in developing nations. As a result, many potential leaders in developing nations are receiving the support and education they need to further address and develop their countries' public health needs.

References

Dale, E. *Audiovisual Methods in Teaching* (3rd. ed.). New York: Dryden Press, 1969.

"Exec-Ed Rankings and Profiles." *Business Week On-line*, Oct. 20, 2003. Available: www.businessweek.com/baschools/03/exc_rank.htm/.

Institute of Medicine. Committee for the Study of the Future of Public Health. *The Future of Public Health.* Washington, D.C.: National Academy Press, 1988.

Institute of Medicine. Committee on Public Health. *Healthy Communities: New Partnerships for the Future of Public Health. A Report of the First Year of the Committee on Public Health.* Washington, D.C.: National Academy Press, 1996.

Walt, G., Pavignani, E., Gilson, L., and Buse, K. "Health Sector Development: From Aid Coordination to Resource Management." *Health Policy and Planning,* 1999, *14*(3), 207–218.

Part V

Leading and Managing Teams
While Recognizing and
Celebrating Success

16

Leading for Success

Nils Daulaire

A leader is best when people barely know he exists,
not so good when people obey and acclaim him,
worse when people despise him.
But of a good leader who talks little when his work is done,
his aim fulfilled, they will say:
We did it ourselves.

Dao De Ching

Disease is simple. A single virulent pathogen, a particular failure of a critical metabolic pathway, a breakdown in a vital aspect of the physical or even social environment, and disease blossoms and spreads. And death is the simplest point on the equation, the unidimensionality of an eternal zero.

In stark contrast, life is infinitely complex. And the fundamental essence of global health—the basis for the continuation of human life on this planet—is that it is the product of a complex system of inputs and processes responding to a wide range of needs, competing demands, and emerging opportunities. For health to be achieved in a way that is both maximal and equitable, for it to cross national borders and social strata, for it to serve as a vehicle of social justice, and for it to incorporate both the technological tools and behavioral changes needed for real impact, all due consideration must be given to this intricate web of connections and interactions.

Appropriate response must mirror the challenges it is designed to address. By its very nature, the complexity of global health cannot effectively be addressed from a single vantage point, no matter how brilliant and committed the practitioner. And experience shows that all truly effective efforts to improve global health have been based on the thoughtful and coordinated work of teams.

Teamwork is often thought about within the context of sports, in which one team competes against another. Unfortunately, this competitive mind-set leads to an exclusivity that works contrary to the goals of better health. In fact, one of the signal aspects of this field is that it is at heart a development process relying on a much wider concept of team, encompassing not only the providers and change agents but also the beneficiaries.

The philosophy underlying this linkage between change agents and those they are trying to serve was perhaps best stated by Ding Xiang (whose anglicized name was James Yen), the founder of the Institute for Rural Reconstruction in China in the first half of the twentieth century. His maxim to those working with him was, "Go to the people, live with the people, learn from the people, plan with the people, work with the people. Start with what they know, build on what they have. Teach by showing, learn by doing. Not a showcase but a pattern, not odds and ends but a system, not piecemeal but an integrated approach. Not to conform but to transform, not relief but release" (Yen, 1960).

What are the characteristics that make teams successful, and how can these be turned toward the mission of promoting better health for all? There are four critical elements:

- Listening

- Learning

- Sharing

- Celebrating

Effective intervention begins with understanding the true nature of the problem, and the reality of ill health is that it is not just a biological issue but also a social issue in both its roots and its effects. Therefore, the first obligation of listening must be to focus on those most affected.

In the 1980s, I worked in Nepal, assisting with the design of health programs directed at children and mothers. In our work in the field, we heard repeatedly from parents that one of their greatest concerns about the well-being of their children was how often they suffered from cough and difficulty breathing. We also knew from epidemiological data that pneumonia was routinely among the leading killers of children under the age of five. Yet, there were no public health programs in place at that time—in Nepal or for that matter, anywhere in the developing world—to address acute respiratory tract infections (ARI) at the community level. And so, listening to those most affected, we set out to do what they had asked.

It turned out that we could learn a lot about intervening in this disease process from listening to mothers. They told us that in rural areas, government hospitals were too distant to serve as major providers of care for issues as widespread and commonplace as ARI, that the more peripheral health posts rarely had drugs available, and that the government staff assigned to both levels of facilities were more often absent than present. So we learned that an effective response would have to be based outside health facilities and to use community-level workers to engage directly with communities.

The mothers told us their indigenous names for this disease and how quickly it developed and worsened, particularly in the very young. Using their descriptions, but applying simple data management tools to what we learned from them, we found that the average time span between the onset of obvious symptoms and death was less than three days. This meant that mothers themselves had to be enlisted as the first-line responders because no realistic scenario could be developed in which all households with young children were visited by our trained community workers every day or two. This would have been necessary to catch most cases in the critical period between clinical manifestation and death.

Listening to those most directly affected was fundamental to the design of the outreach intervention we developed. But effective leadership goes beyond listening to the client. The essence of a team is not simply that it provides a multiplicity of hands to carry out work but that it also provides a multiplicity of eyes and ears to see reality from a variety of vantage points and a multiplicity of brains to provide insights and reflection. All too often, management is manifested in a "command-and-control" mentality that makes inadequate use—or no use at all—of these resources. Yet, the history of the quality improvement movement that revolutionized business in the last part of the twentieth century was based on the premise that every person along the chain of production has the potential to add value and efficiency to the process and that the mark of an effective manager (and, I would add, leader) is to solicit, listen to, and act on this input.

One of the first companies to refine this process was Toyota, which became known globally as the automotive manufacturer with the highest quality for price and the lowest variability in quality from car to car. Notably, Toyota empowered its line workers not only to make suggestions for improvements but to actually shut down the assembly line if problems were discovered that called for a systemic response.

Likewise, in Nepal we learned to rely on the insights of our "line workers," the community health agents. Although barely literate, many with no more than a few years of formal schooling, these workers knew their communities intimately. Based on their feedback, we modified house-visiting schedules, developed more appropriate health-education materials, refined our case-detection training as we added new agents, and simplified our systems for maintaining and resupplying antibiotic stocks. And in turn, because they were empowered in ways that gave them a real sense of ownership of the program, they continued to work at times when funding gaps made it impossible to continue even their nominal payments, and they assumed responsibility for making sure that their communities were served when political conditions during Nepal's Maoist uprising forced an end to the formal program. In this as in so many other cases, listening to and engaging staff was perhaps the most important element of sustainability.

But listening has limited value without continuous learning, and learning must come from external as well as internal sources, or efforts run the risk of becoming exclusively self-referential. As global health practitioners, we have the obligation to use the tools of biomedical and behavioral sciences and the rigorous discipline of epidemiology to assure that what we are doing is of maximal potential value to those we intend to serve. Unfortunately, the world is replete with often well-meaning efforts to improve health that have not undergone the internal scrutiny that learning requires.

In Nepal, for instance, we were able to learn based on a review of public health literature that recent hospital-based studies in Papua–New Guinea had shown that the use of respiratory rate and the visible presence of substernal and intercostal retractions (chest in-drawing) provided an adequately reliable basis for the diagnosis of pneumonia. From studies carried out in Pakistan, we learned that, in marked contrast to clinical experience in hospitals in the United States, the large majority of cases of serious pneumonia with high risk of mortality in poor communities were the result of bacterial infections and amenable to treatment with relatively inexpensive first-line antibiotics. We therefore had the scientific basis for a premise: that the community health agents we had trained would be in a position to actually diagnose and treat pneumonia in the community.

However, learning is not possible without an honest assessment of failures and successes; every failure should be seen as an opportunity to assess, modify, and improve. Unfortunately, this rule is often abandoned in the efforts by some global health programs to attract and keep resources and the mistaken impression by some that leadership means "never having to say you're sorry."

In Nepal, we learned, for instance, that our initial complicated data collection system, intended to provide a sensitive barometer for case-detection rates, was such a recording and reporting burden to the agents that it served as an impediment to effective work rather than as an aid. This burden also actually reduced the accuracy of reporting, introducing so much noise to the system that it could not serve its initial purpose. The agents complained and suggested simplifications, the leadership listened and learned, and we dropped some study aspects for the sake of better efficacy. Similarly, when early in the program our data showed no significant change in child mortality despite evidence that agents were adhering to protocol, we looked for reasons that we might be failing even if the underlying concept was right. That was when we learned that visiting households on a two-week schedule was unlikely to connect with most children suffering from pneumonia because of the rapid course of the disease and, as noted above, we enlisted mothers as our actual front-line workers.

Every successful global health program is replete with failures of this sort that have been identified and addressed. None of us is smart enough to figure out the possible obstacles and confounders in advance, and the mark of true leadership is the willingness to approach these questions with humility and honesty.

But implementing a successful program is not enough. Sharing—expanding impact beyond the initial population served—is an essential component of global health leadership. Just as the early ARI studies in Papua–New Guinea and Pakistan shared their knowledge with us, we looked to share our experiences and learning with others working to improve child health. Initially this sharing took place at the closest concentric circle. Once it became clear from our studies that this approach to community-based care of ARI had a significant effect on childhood mortality, we shared our findings and experiences with other health programs working in Nepal and also with the ministry of health. With proof of the concept in hand, this provided the basis over the ensuing decade for Nepal to expand ARI case management to virtually the entire country. As of the time of this writing, Nepal, despite its political problems, is considered one of the world's model countries in pneumonia control.

With evidence of the role of mothers in this process, national policy was redirected toward the development and support of female community health volunteers, who had the best access to these mothers, as first-line workers. With the validation of antibiotic use by trained nonphysicians, the government modified its regulations concerning who was allowed to dispense first-line antibiotics. Nationally, Nepal has witnessed a dramatic decline in its under-five mortality during this period.

But this issue, as with most in the field of global health, was not restricted to one community or nation. Sharing also requires going to the widest possible audience so that others may take and modify what has been learned for their own needs. With the publication of our findings in 1991 (Pandey and others) and the adoption by the World Health Organization and the United Nations Children's Fund of the standard ARI case-management protocol as the appropriate first-level response to pneumonia at the community level, the approach that took root in a remote district of Nepal two decades ago has become a global standard. This was driven home to me recently when I visited a rural clinic in the highlands of Honduras, literally half a world away from Nepal. There I found trained community health agents using virtually the same protocol we had field-tested, going door-to-door to detect and treat pneumonia in young children.

The most dramatic examples of leadership in global health have taken the approach of listening, learning, and sharing. Among these are the first four winners of the U.S.\$1 million Gates Award for Global Health, considered by some the Nobel Prize of the twenty-first century. The Bangladesh Center for Health and Population Research (of the International Center for Diarrheal Disease Research of Bangladesh, or ICDDRB)—lauded by Melinda French Gates in an earlier chapter of this book—carried out the basic and applied research to develop oral rehydration therapy and to show what it would take to reduce global deaths from childhood diarrhea. Rotary International demonstrated the power of committed communities from outside the health arena to make an impact on a global disease, polio, to generate vast new resources for global health and to lead to the eradication of an age-old virus. The Brazilian National AIDS (acquired immunodeficiency syndrome) Program showed that governments that take seriously their responsibilities to the health of their most vulnerable, that are not afraid to challenge either public prejudice or private interests, and that integrate prevention and care in a systematic approach to this plague can indeed roll back the AIDS pandemic. And BRAC (formerly the Bangladesh Rural Advancement Committee) has demonstrated all of the attributes of global health leadership discussed in this chapter: a community-based approach not simply to health but to economic development, empowerment of women, and education that has lifted the lives of tens of millions of Bangladeshis out of poverty and ill health and served as the model for nongovernmental organizations working throughout the developing world.

But what of celebrating? Where does this enter into the picture of global health leadership?

In each of the cases I have cited, celebration has been an integral part of what has kept the process on track. Ultimately, every global health program rests on the energy and commitment of the people struggling to make it work. This is hardly a well-remunerated field, so motivation cannot come from the financial arena. The complications and setbacks are innumerable, and the realities are that for every two steps forward, we often experience a step-and-a-half back, so the short feedback loops of success and validation are generally not available to us. No, for the most part, the validation and motivation that keep people working, listening, learning, and sharing toward this common goal come from the sense of community that these successful programs have been able to instill.

Community is a fundamental concept based on shared values and a common vision. Leadership plays a critical role in helping to identify and verbalize both. But these are not enough to maintain community in the face of continuous obstacles and adversity. Celebration is a common thread in all communities and a fundamental need of the human psyche. It is expressed in ways small and large.

In each of the programs I have mentioned, leaders have taken the time—have, in fact, made a priority—of instilling a sense of celebration for advances made. Public recognition of performance by engendering internal groups that could provide support and encouragement, joint community activities that had color as well as effect, and a continuous effort to revisit original questions and view every step of the learning process as the occasion for joy is a common thread of well-led programs. Once instilled and quietly supported, often these have then been carried out without the visible presence of the leaders who established them.

Celebration takes place both on a global scale and on a small scale. This was the premise underlying the decision by the Bill and Melinda Gates Foundation to establish the Gates Award for Global Health. The U.S.$1 million prize is not based on a proposal for work that is planned; it is not a grant restricted to a particular aspect of the winner's activities or in any way directed from the outside. Rather, it serves as the crown jewel of celebration for contribution to the health of the world's least fortunate, a recognition of substantial and lasting effects on global health.

In a fundamental way, it is what each successful leader does on a daily basis, in ways large and small, showing that the efforts undertaken on behalf of health improvement and equity are meaningful and important and that each contribution, no matter how small, is meaningful and important in itself. It states that it is the steady work that matters, not the occasional celebrity spotlight.

For every one of the recipients of the Gates Award, and for those whose work on the front lines has led to this recognition and celebration, the quiet refrain echoes in their heads: we did it ourselves.

References

Pandey, M. R., and others. "Reduction in Total Under-Five Mortality in Western Nepal Through Community-Based Antimicrobial Treatment of Pneumonia." *Lancet*, 1991, *338*, 993–997.

Yen, Y. C. James, Institute for Rural Reconstruction, 1960. Available: www.irr.org/valuescredo.html.

17

Epilogue
The Road Ahead

Kofi A. Annan

In 2000, the largest-ever gathering of world leaders came together to adopt the Millennium Development Goals, a blueprint for building a better world in the twenty-first century. The goals express a set of simple but powerful objectives that every man and woman in the street, from New York to Nairobi to New Delhi, can easily support and understand. Health is explicit in some of them: reducing child mortality, improving maternal health, halting the spread of human immunodeficiency virus (HIV), malaria, and other communicable diseases, and implicit in the others: reducing poverty, empowering women, ensuring environmental sustainability, and achieving universal primary education.

As the Millennium Development Goals indicate, we know that health is a prerequisite for development. Leadership for health must come from every level of society, from the health worker with the megaphone telling her community about an immunization campaign to the scientists determining how to minimize the global risk of the next flu pandemic, from the nurse providing voluntary counseling on HIV/AIDS (acquired immunodeficiency syndrome) to the governments and donors who determine priorities in the allocation of resources. Qualified people are essential, and urgent investment in the right training, particularly in the developing world, is crucial to our ability to attain the Millennium Development Goals. We also need to ensure that health systems in every country can serve all people, whoever and wherever they are, rural and urban, rich and poor, and provide a broad range of care, whether for expectant mothers, their newborn children, or their grandparents.

Achieving this requires leadership and responsibility among donor and recipient governments alike. It requires us to work in partnership—between the developed and developing world, among governments, international organizations, civil society, and the private sector.

That is why the Millennium Development Goals are so valuable. They are a tool both for mobilizing support and for holding governments accountable. They represent a call to action and a way of keeping track of the results that matter most: building better, healthier lives for people across the planet. It is a call to which the world can and must respond. Reaching the goals, however, does not mean reaching the end. As a deadline for meeting a set of minimum standards, the Millennium Development Goals represent a milestone in our continuing work toward global equity in the provision of public health.

Index

A

AARP (formerly American Association of Retired Persons), 39, 40, 42
Abbott Laboratories, 18
ABIA (Associação Brasileira Interdisciplinar de AIDS) [Brazil], 78, 79, 90
Abrahamson, D., 57
Accelerating Access Initiative, 18
Action learning model, 207, 208
Adany, R., 175
Aging population: benefits of healthy aging by, 47; challenges of, 39–40; growing health expenditures spent on, 41; long-term care/disease management and, 43–44; percentage of workers among, 47; public policies on "frail elderly" of, 58. *See also* Longevity/life expectancy
AIDS. *See* HIV/AIDS
Akunyili, D., 99, 100
Alexander, D., 45
American Cancer Society: accomplishments through collaboration by, 142–143; C-Change partnership formed by, 134, 135–137; collaboration embraced by, 131–132; collaboration lessons learned by, 139–142; OVAC (One Voice Against Cancer) formed by, 137–139; partnerships ended into by, 134; Preventive Health Partnership of, 143; quality standards for collaboration followed by, 132–133
American College of Surgeons, 134
American Diabetes Association, 43, 143
American Heart Association, 143
Andreev, E. M., 168, 171
Andrija Stampar School of Public Health (Croatia), 173, 181
Anell, A., 150
Annan, K. A., 6, 115, 227
Anticorruption: civil society supporting, 99–100; industry partnerships promoting, 97–99; NIS (National Integrity System) approach to, 96–97; as pro-global health, 100–101. *See also* Corruption
ARI (acute respiratory tract infections), 219, 222–223
Aristotle, 66
ARVs (antiretroviral drugs): Brazilian negotiations to reduce prices of, 85, 86–87; Brazilian program providing/tracking free, 76, 87–89; as breakthrough discovery, 84; donor support for providing, 150; high price of, 75; "3-by-5" initiative on, 29, 31–32, 35, 193–194

arznei-telegramm (independent German drugs bulletin), 99
ASPHER (Association of Schools of Public Health in the European Region), 175, 182
AZT (zidovudine), 84

B
Badouy, J., 149
Bangalore (India), 93–94
Basic human needs: difficulty of defining categories of, 60–61; interlocked complexity of, 59; types of, 60
Basic Human Needs report (1978), 61
Belicza, B., 173
Bennett, S., 151
Beveridge, W., 32, 34
Bhattacharya, J., 46
Bill and Melinda Gates Foundation. *See* Gates Foundation
Bill and Melinda Gates Institute for Population and Reproductive Health, 211
Biz/AIDS program: development of, 107–111; origins of, 105–106; three tiers of, 106–107
Boehringer-Ingelheim, 18
Bojan, F., 172, 174, 175
Borovecki, A., 173
Bosma, H., 171
Botswana-Merck-Gates Foundation partnership, 10–11, 15, 19, 20. *See also* Merck
Boufford, J. I., 147
BP, 98
BRAC (formerly Bangladesh Rural Advancement Committee), 224
Brazilian HIV/AIDS epidemic: free ARVs program, 75, 76, 84, 85, 86–89; future of Brazilian approach to, 89–91; government response to, 78–83; government-sponsored treatment of, 83–89; role of NGOs in response to, 78–79, 82; unique and successful approach to, 75–78
BRIMHEALTH program, 177

Bristol-Myers Squibb, 18
Browne, Lord J., 22
Brundtland, G. H., 59
Bruno, G., 170
Buch, E., 151
"Building and Maintaining Advocacy Coalitions" (Schultz), 130
Bury, J., 181
Buse, K., 155, 202
"Business Principles for Countering Bribery" website, 98–99
Business sector. *See* Corporate America

C
C=Change (National Dialogue on Cancer): function/purpose of, 134; organization/strategies used by, 136–137; seven principles followed by, 135
CamCare project (Netherlands), 48
Campaign for Tobacco-Free Kids, 39
Camus, A., 34
CARE, 49
Carter Center, 16
Cash, R. A., 154
Cavallo, F., 181
Cazazu, A., 172
CDC (Centers for Disease Control and Prevention): American Cancer Society partnership with, 134; OVAC efforts to increase funding for, 138; public health leadership development role by, 204; reporting on chronic diseases, 43; supporting investments in public health systems leadership, 156; Sustainable Management Development Program of, 156, 210–211
Celebration, 218, 225
Center for Health and Population Research (Bangladesh), 7–8
Central Europe: creating public health leadership in, 173–176; developing health career opportunities in, 178–179; health legacy in, 172–173; longevity/life expectancy

in, 168; positive impact of public health in, 180–181; securing long-term funding for public health in, 179–180; successful health collaboration in, 181–182; successful health programs in, 177–178

Change agents, 218

Change teams: critical elements of successful, 218; effective intervention using, 219; examples of interventions by, 219–225

Chapman, S., 181

Chen, L. C., 154

Chenet, L., 172

Chief Executive (magazine), 157

Childhood diarrhea, 7–8, 224

Children: impact of structural adjustment programs on, 193; life benefits of healthy behaviors by, 45–46; percentage of overweight, 46

Chisholm, B., 25

Cholera epidemic (London, 1849), 129, 143

Cipla (Indian drug manufacturer), 86

Civil society: anticorruption efforts by, 93–94, 99–100; health investments supported by, 118; needs assessment to appreciate, 188–189. *See also* NGOs (nongovernmental organizations)

Cleveland, H., 55, 59, 61

CMH (Commission on Macroeconomics and Health), 115, 116–117

Coca-Cola Africa Foundation, 21

Coca-Cola Company, 21

Colatella, B. D., 10

Collaborations. *See* Global health partnerships; Public health alliances

Collaborative leadership, 158

Comim, F., 179

Commission on Education for Public Health (U.S.), 203–204

Commission on Macroeconomics and Health, 151

Community concept, 225

Computer-assisted communication, 62–64

The Constant Gardener (Le CarrÈ), 94, 100

Cope, M. K., 105, 109

Copernicus, 169, 170

Copperlink Program (IESC), 108, 109

Corporate America: anticorruption partnerships with, 97–99; Botswana-Merck-Gates Foundation partnership, 10–11, 15, 19, 20; comprehensive health programs/partnerships by, 12–15; global economy and social challenges role of, 9–10; improving global health as imperative of, 11–12; leadership development in, 157–158; pharmaceutical companies, 85, 86–87, 99–100; re-evaluating NGO involvement with, 21–22; response to HIV/AIDS by, 17–23; taking the time to study health needs, 13; value of workings with NGOs, 13–14

Corporate Council on Africa, 22

Corruption: impact on health care services, 93–94; "pharma-marketing," 99–100; unhealthy world order due to, 94–96. *See also* Anticorruption

Critical Issues, 56, 64, 70

Crixivan (indinivir sulfate), 17

Croatia, 173, 181

Czech Republic, 180, 211

D

DaimlerChrysler, 20–21

Dale, E., 206

DANIDA (Danish International Development Agency), 150

Dao De Ching, 217

Daulaire, N., 64, 217

DDT spraying, 25, 26

Declaration of Alma-Ata (WHO), 38

Democracy Owners Manual (Schultz), 130

Denisov, I., 176

Dentzer, S., 75

DeSalle, R., 129

Developing countries: CMH estimates on cost of basic health services in, 115; health investments in, 115–117; implementation gap in, 148, 162–163; inadequate health infrastructures in, 147; inadequate health services/poverty link in, 48; information gap of, 67–68; leadership development for health systems in, 151–153, 202–203; leadership development programs in, 209–213; Monterrey Consensus (2002) signed by, 114–115; "participation gap" of, 154–155; PRSPs (Poverty Reduction Strategy Papers) submitted by, 118. *See also* Poverty

DfID (Department for International Development) [UK], 150

Dhaka hospital (Bangladesh), 8

Diabetes, 43–44

Ding Xiang, 218

Diseases: ARI (acute respiratory tract infections), 219, 222–223; childhood diarrhea, 7–8, 224; diabetes, 43–44; "double burden" of chronic and infectious, 59; malaria, 12; management of, 43–44; river blindness (onchocerciasis), 16; SARS (severe acute respiratory syndrome), 9, 38, 189; smallpox eradication campaign (1970s), 32. *See also* HIV/AIDS

Doctors Without Borders, 49

Dolea, C., 168

Downs, A. M., 168

Drayer, N., 155

Drucker, P., 71, 124, 125

Dubos, R., 57

E

Eastern Europe: creating public health leadership in, 173–176; developing health career opportunities in, 178–179; health legacy in, 172–173; health status/morality rates in, 167–169; positive impact of public health in, 180–181; securing long-term funding for public health in, 179–180; successful health collaboration in, 181–182; successful health programs in, 177–178

Ebola virus-causes hemorrhagic fever, 38

The Economist (magazine), 63–64, 124

Edna McConnell Clark Foundation, 17

Eigen, P., 93

Eklund, L., 177

"Elite pluralism" phenomenon, 155

Emerging Leaders in Public Health program (U.S.), 205–206

Emery, C. F., 46

Emilio Ribas hospital (Sao Paolo, Brazil), 80

Emory University (Atlanta), 176

Engels, F., 169

Enhancing Care Initiative (Harvard School of Public Health), 17–18

Epidemiologic Intelligence Service, 156

Equity issues, 155

EU (European Union), 49

EUPHA (European Public Health Association), 175, 182

European Commission, 41

European Public Health Alliance, 182

Evang, K., 26

Evans, T. G., 154

Expanded Program on Immunization, 32

F

F. Hoffmann-la Roche, 18

Fairness revolution, 64–68

Family size, 49

Feacham, R.G.A., 154

FETP (Field Epidemiology Training Program), 156

Field, M. G., 170
Filerman, G., 70
Fiocruz (Oswaldo Cruz Foundation)
    [Brazil], 84–85
Foege, W. H., 59
Fogarty Center (National Institutes
    of Health), 156–157
Fogarty Fellowship, 209
Former Soviet Union: declining life
    expectancy rates in, 167, 168;
    health legacy of the past in, 169;
    mortality rates in, 167–168; secur-
    ing long-term public health funding
    for, 180; Soviet science of, 169–172
Francois-Xavier Bagnoud Center
    (Harvard School of Public Health),
    17–18
Freedom to grow up, 4
Freedoms, 3–4
Freeman, B., 22
Fuseon, 88
Fustkian, S., 155
The Future of Public Health (IOM),
    203

G
G8 countries, 27
Galen, 169
Gallup, J. L., 12
Garner, P., 154
Gates Award for Global Health, 3, 7,
    76, 223, 225
Gates, B., 5
Gates Foundation: creation and
    global health focus of, 4, 5;
    HIV/AIDS program partnership
    (Botswana) by, 10–11, 15, 19, 20
Gates Institute for Population and
    Reproductive Health, 211
Gates, M. F., 3, 223
GDP (gross domestic product): Brazil-
    ian, 77; health expenditures as per-
    centage of, 40, 192
General Electric, 98, 157
Generalist health leadership, 71–73
Gilead, 18

Gillies, P., 131
Gilmartin, R. V., 9
Gilmore, A., 181
Gilson, L., 202
Gjonca, A., 172
GlaxoSmithKline, Inc., 17, 18, 88,
    95–96
Glenngård, A., 150
Global Alliance for TB Drug Devel-
    opment, 98
Global Business Coalition on
    HIV/AIDS, 21
Global fairness revolution, 64–68
Global Fund to Fight AIDS, Tubercu-
    losis and Malaria, 27, 118
Global health: action as source of ideas
    to promote, 32–35; anticorruption
    as pro, 100–101; Botswana-Merck-
    Gates Foundation partnership to
    improve, 10–11; business impera-
    tive/strategies to improve, 11–15;
    challenges of, 39–44, 123–125,
    189–198; corporate America's
    role in, 9–23; expectations of,
    125–126; fundamental essence
    of, 217; health management to
    improve, 56–59; leadership devel-
    opment for, 153–155; reality
    check regarding status of, 4; as
    required for global stability, 6;
    teams/teamwork used to improve,
    218–225; technology perceived as
    solution to, 25; three gaps in public
    policymaking on, 154–155. See also
    Health; Public health
Global health challenges: appropriate
    response mirroring the, 218; faced
    by leadership, 123–125; framework
    for addressing, 190–195; global per-
    spective of, 197–198; increased
    longevity and aging population,
    39–40; increasing health expendi-
    tures/access as, 40–43; local context
    of, 189–190; long-term care/disease
    management as, 43–44; people-
    centered approach to, 195–197

Global Health Council (GHC), 5

Global Health Council to the Global Business Coalition on HIV/AIDS, 22

Global health gap, 191

Global health leadership: art of principled, 126–128; challenges faced by, 123–125, 189–190; community concept as identified/verbalized by, 225; development of, 151–164, 173–182, 187–199; framework for addressing health issues by, 190–195; generalist, 71–73; global perspective of, 197–198; health needs goals of, 125–126; need for global collaboration and, 48–50; needs assessment by, 187–189; nobody in charge model of, 69–71; opportunities for, 44–48; people-centered approach used by, 195–197; "planned abandonment" task of, 125; redefining, 127; shifting from vertical to horizontal, 68. *See also* Health systems; Public health leadership institutes

Global health leadership development: in Central/Eastern Europe, 173–182; in developing countries, 151–153, 202–203, 209–213; at the global level, 153–155; model for, 155–161*fig*; need for, 151; in the United States, 203–209

Global health partnerships: agreement on shared set of goals, 14; benefits of creating strong, 12–15; Botswana-Merck-Gates Foundation, 10–11, 15; in Central and Eastern Europe, 181–182; focusing on the long term, 14–15; four types of, 30–32; public health, 129–143; securing high-level commitment/engagement, 14; transparency as required in, 15; two decades of lessons learned through, 15–17; value of assembling broad range of partners for, 13–14. *See also* Public health alliances

Goldman, D. P., 46

Gordon, D. F., 12

"Great man theory," 158

Green Revolution (1970s) [India], 67

Gribbin, J., 169

Grunberg, I., 154

GTZ (Germany), 20

H

Hadassah School of Public Health (Jerusalem), 176

Hamers, F. F., 168

Handy, C. B., 183

Harvard AIDS Institute, 17

Harvard School of Public Health, 210

Health: increased longevity and, 38; longevity as measurement of population, 61; poverty and poor, 64; progressive nature of, 38–39; UN Declaration of Human Rights on right to, 60. *See also* Global health; Public health

Health for all model, 33, 38, 198

Health behaviors: adult afflictions originating in childhood, 45; benefits of good, 45; changing to improve, 46–47; as form of self-management, 56–59; global efforts to improve, 47–48; impact of obesity, 45–46

Health expenditures: aging population and growth in, 41; challenge of finding innovative solutions to, 42–43; European vs. American differences regarding, 41–42; GDP percentage spent on, 40, 192; morality rates tied to, 192–193; U.S. Veterans Health Administration's approach to, 48

Health management: global fairness revolution and, 64–68; information revolution and, 62–64; potential health improvements through, 56–57

Health Resources and Services Administration, 134

Health services: CMH estimates on cost of delivering basic, 115; combating corruption impacting, 93–101; investments in developing countries to increase, 115–117; relationship between poverty and inadequate, 48

Health systems: future steps for leadership development in, 161–164; human resources for, 148–150; implementation gap in developing countries, 148; model for leadership development in, 155–161; need for leadership development for, 151–155, 202–203. *See also* Global health leadership

Health-for-all movement (1980s), 32

Healthy aging benefits, 47

Healthy Communities: New Partnerships for the Future of Public Health (IOM report), 203

Healy, J., 173

Henry J. Kaiser Family Foundation, 77

Hesselbein, F., 123, 124

Hierarchies of countries, 68–69

HIV/AIDS: ARVs (antiretroviral drugs) treatment of, 75, 76, 84, 85, 86–89, 150; behavioral change interventions lagging for, 191; benefits of assembling partners in fighting, 14; Botswana-Merck-Gates Foundation partnership to fight, 10–11, 15, 19, 20; Brazilian approach to, 75–91; corporate America's response to, 17–23; demoralization due to, 193; estimates on people living with, 28–29; global fight against, 6–7, 26–27; IESC's business approach to combating, 103–111; as new evolutionary step, 59; rapid worldwide spread of, 12, 26–27, 28; rising rates of Soviet Union, 168; Romanian epidemic of, 172; taking the time to study communities and state of, 13;

"3-by-5" initiative to combat, 29, 31–32, 35, 193–194; twenty-first century initiative to combat, 27–32. *See also* Diseases

"HIV/AIDS in the Workplace" program (IESC), 108–109

Hoffmann-La Roche, 18

House of Hope (Botswana), 10

Hubert H. Humphrey Fellowship program, 209

"Human Genome Survey" (*The Economist*), 63–64

Hungary, 174–176, 175, 211

I

ICDDR,B (International Center for Diarrhea Disease Research, Bangladesh), 7–8, 223–224

IESC (International Executive Service Corps): approach to HIV/AIDS crisis by, 104–105; background of, 103–104; Copperlink Program of, 108, 109; development of Biz/AIDS process, 107–111; "HIV/AIDS in the Workplace" program of, 108–109; Livingstone Linkages program of USAID and, 108; SABCOHA proposal by, 110, 111; *SME Business Survival Planning Workbook* (2004) of, 109; Zambia's Biz/AIDS programs under, 105–107

Immunization, 59

Implementation gap, 148, 162–163

India's Green Revolution (1970s), 67

Infant mortality rates, 167–168, 192–193

Information: computer-assisted communication of, 62–64; expansion during use of, 62; fairness revolution and distribution of, 64–68; free public education and, 66–67; global impact of, 62; as new dominant resource/hierarchy, 68–69; poverty/wealth and, 67–68

Institute of Medicine (IOM), 203

Institute for Rural Reconstruction (China), 218
International AIDS Conference (1996, Vancouver), 84
International Center for Creative Leadership development programs, 206
International Conference on Financing for Development, 114
International Monetary Fund, 118
IntraHealth International, 212

J

JLI (Joint Learning Initiative) [Rockefeller Foundation], 148–150, 162
Johns Hopkins University, 210
Johnson & Johnson, 211
Johnson, N., 158, 162
Jong-wook, L., 25
Jorasvsky, D., 170

K

Kalediene, R., 177
Kalichman, A., 81, 83, 89
Kaul, I., 154
Kaunas-Rotterdam heart disease study, 171
Keusch, G., 157
King, S. T., 103
Kohler, L., 177
Kozinetz, C., 172
Krementosov, N. L., 169

L

Lakdawalla, D. N., 46
Larson, C., 155
Law/fairness link, 66
Le CarrÈ, J., 94
Leadership development. See Global health leadership development
Leadership for Global Health (Office of Public Management), 161
Leadership. See Global health leadership
Lee, K., 155

Leite, G. S., 82
Lenin, V., 169
Lepeshinskkaia, O., 170
Leppo, K., 149
Listening, 218, 221–222, 223
Livingstone Linkages program (IESC-USAID), 108
London School of Hygiene and Tropical Medicine, 177
Long-term care, 43–44
Longevity/life expectancy: in Central Europe, 168; challenges of increased, 39–40; declining rates in former Soviet Union, 167, 168; global gains in, 38; as measuring population's health, 61; social value of, 58–59. See also Aging population
"Looking Ahead" (Pearson and Filerman), 70
"Lula" (Luiz Inacio Lula da Silva), 90
Lysenko, T., 170

M

McHale, J., 60, 61
McHale, M., 60, 61
McKee, M., 154, 167, 168, 171, 172, 173, 174, 175
McMichael, A. J., 168
Malaria, 12
Mandela, N., 5, 6
Matusa, R., 172
Marusic, A., 181
Marx, K., 169
Maternal mortality rates, 167–168, 192
MDGs (Millennium Development Goals): described, 227–228; global mobilization to reach, 148; on health investments in developing countries, 115–116; regarding developing countries, 113–114; strategies to attain, 116–118. See also United Nations
Medicaid, 43–44
Medicare, 43–44

Melum, M., 157
Merck: ARV global pricing policy
  of, 86; Brazilian ARV negotiations
  with, 85; corporate responsibility
  efforts by, 10–11, 12, 15, 18, 23;
  river blindness treatment collabora-
  tion with WHO, 16, 17. *See also*
  Botswana-Merck-Gates Foundation
  partnership
Merck Company Foundation, 19
Merck, G. W., 98
Merck Mectizan Donation Program,
  10, 13, 15, 16–17
Milen, A., 149
Millennium Development Goals
  (UN declaration), 27
Mills, A., 151
Mills, G., 154, 155
"Mission creep" potential, 15
Model for leadership development,
  155–161*fig*
Mogae, F., 10
MONICA program (WHO), 171
Monterrey Consensus (2002),
  114–115
Morality rates: in former Soviet
  Union, 167–168; health expendi-
  tures tied to, 192–193
Morrill Act (1862), 67
Moscow Medical Academy, 176, 177
MSH (Management Sciences for
  Health), 212
Munhoz, R., 88–89
Musgrove, P., 33
Myers, J., 45

N

Naidoo, K., 56
Nalliah, V., 26
National Cancer Act (1971), 132
National Cancer Institute, 132, 134,
  138, 139
National Center on Minority Health
  and Health Disparities, 138
National Comprehensive Cancer
  Network, 134

National Institutes of Health, 45, 138
National Public Health Leadership
  Institute (PHLI), 156, 204–205
NBCAM (National Breast Cancer
  Awareness Month), 142
Needle-exchange programs, 80, 81
Nepal health programs, 219–221, 222
Neufeld, V., 158, 162
New England Journal of Medicine, 45
New Partnership for African Development, 151
The NewsHour with Jim Lehrer (PBS),
  77
NGOs (nongovernmental organizations): anticorruption efforts by,
  93–94, 99–100; global health
  expectations of, 125; health system
  leadership within, 203; HIV/AIDS
  program partnerships of corpora-
  tions and, 21; re-evaluating corpo-
  rate involvement with, 21–22; role
  in Brazil's response to HIV/AIDS,
  78–79, 82; as suspicious of corporate motives, 19; value of working
  with, 13–14. *See also* Civil society
Nigeria's National Agency for Food
  and Drug Administration and Control, 99
NIS (National Integrity System),
  96–97
Nobody in charge model, 69–71
Nolte, E., 168
"Nomadic quotations," 169–170
NORAD (Norwegian Agency for
  International Development), 150
Nordic School of Public Health, 177
Normand, C., 181
Norsk Hydro, 98
Novartis, 98
Novelli, W., 37

O

Obesity, 45–46
OECD (Organization for Economic
  Cooperation and Development),
  40, 41, 49, 67

Office of Public Management, 158, 160, 161

Ohio State University study (2003), 46

Onchocerciasis (river blindness), 16, 17

The One Minute Manager, 72

Open Society Institute (Soros Foundation), 176, 178, 182

Orešković, S., 173

ORS (oral rehydration solution), 7–8, 224

Ostbye, T., 172, 175

Osteoporosis, 45

Oswaldo Cruz Foundation (Brazil), 84–85

OVAC (One Voice Against Cancer), 137–139

P

Padayachee, N., 10

Pakistan, 221, 222

Pandey, M. R., 223

Papua-New Guinea, 222

"Participation gap," 154–155

Partnerships. *See* Global health partnerships; Public health alliances

Pavignani, E., 202

Pearson, C., 70

Pediatric Clinics of America, 46

People-centered leadership approach, 195–197

Pfizer, 17

Pharmaceutical companies: Brazilian ARVs negotiations with, 85, 86–87; "pharma-marketing" corruption by, 99–100

Phillips, J., 158

PHLI (National Public Health Leadership Institute), 156, 204–205

Phumaphi, J., 187

Pimenta, C., 78, 79, 90, 91

Pinheiro, G., 76–77, 91

Pinheiro, M., 77

The Plague (Camus), 34

"Planned abandonment" task, 125

Pope, A., 39

Porter, J., 201

Porter, R., 25

Poverty: information gap and, 67–68; MDGs (Millennium Development Goals) to reduce, 113–114; poor health as function of, 64; relationship between inadequate health services and, 48. *See also* Developing countries

Powell, C., 6

Powles, J. W., 168, 179

Preventive Health Partnership, 143

Principled leadership, 126–128

Procter & Gamble, 97

Project Hope (Johnson & Johnson), 211

Prostitution Civil Rights and Health (Brazil), 82

PRSPs (Poverty Reduction Strategy Papers), 118

Ptolemy, 169

Public Affairs Center website, 93

Public health: creating Central and Eastern European leadership for, 173–178; creating Russian leadership for, 176–177; development in Hungary, 174–176. *See also* Global health; Health

Public health alliances: C=Change experience with, 135–137; future of collaboration and, 142–143; lessons learned about, 139–142; making collaboration an organizational priority in, 131–134; OVAC (One Voice Against Cancer) experience with, 137–139; reviewing literature on, 130–131. *See also* Global health partnerships

Public health leadership institutes: in developing countries, 209–213; development of U.S., 203–209; need for, 201–202. *See also* Global health leadership

R

Ramalingaswami, Professor, 59

Rao, M., 155

Red Cross, 49
Reflection learning model, 207–208
Rimpela, A., 181
River blindness (onchocerciasis),
    16, 17
Rockefeller Foundation, 173
Rockefeller Foundation JLI (Joint
    Learning Initiative), 148–150, 162
Romania, 172, 180
Roosevelt, E., 60
Roosevelt, F. D., 3
Roper, W. L., 201
Russell, S., 151
Russia, 167, 168, 176–177

S
SABCOHA (South Africa Business
    Coalition on HIV/AIDS), 110, 111
Sachs, J. D., 12, 48, 113, 147, 151, 154
SARS (severe acute respiratory syn-
    drome), 9, 38, 189
Schlaiss, K.-H., 21
Sch^nh^fer, P. S., 99–100
Schultz, J., 130
Schwattlander, B., 29
Seffrin, J. R., 129
Sctliff, R., 156
Shell, 98
Sherman, J., 109
Shkolnikov, V. M., 168
SIDA (Swedish International Devel-
    opment Agency), 150
Smallpox eradication campaign
    (1970s), 32
SME Business Survival Planning Work-
    book (2004) [IESC], 109
SMEs (small and medium enterprises)
    [Zambia], 106, 107, 110, 111
Smoking dangers, 46
Snow, J., 129
Social Accountability International,
    98
"Social Insurance and Allied Ser-
    vices" (Beveridge report), 32–33
Soros Foundation (Open Society
    Institute), 176, 178, 182

Southeast Public Health Leadership
    Institute, 205
Soviet science, 169–172
Soyfer, V. N., 170
Spain, 181
Spiro, L. N., 157
Stalin, J., 169
Stampar, A., 173
Stern, M. A., 154
Stiglitz, J. E., 155
Stocrin (efavirenz), 17
Stott, R., 154
Structural adjustment programs,
    192–193
Sturchio, J. L., 10
Sustainable Management Develop-
    ment Program (CDC), 156,
    210–211
Syncor International Corporation, 95
Syncor Taiwan, 95

T
Tagore, R., 8
Tata, 98
Teams. See Change teams
Technological advances: benefits
    of communication and transporta-
    tion, 37; impact of computer/
    telecommunications, 62–63; impact
    on global leadership of health sys-
    tems, 153; perceived as solution
    to health problems, 25; related to
    information, 62–64; of Soviet sci-
    ence, 169–172
Teixeira, P., 79–80, 82, 84, 89
Teixeira, R. B., 80
Thompson, T., 82
"3-by-5" initiative, 29, 31–32, 35,
    193–194
TI Integrity Award, 99
TI (Transparency International),
    94, 98, 99, 100
TI's Bribe Payers' Survey 2002, 95
Tkatchenko, E., 171
Tobacco use, 46
Tokin, B. P., 170

Toyota, 220
Traubel, H., 7
Tsouros, A. D., 171
Tulchinsky, T., 176
Tunstall-Pedoe, H., 171
Turning Point Leadership Development National Excellence Collaborative in the United States, 155
Twilight of hierarchy, 68–69

U

U.K.'s National Health Service, 33
U.N. Environmental Program, 61
U.N. Population Fund, 18
UNAIDS (Joint United Nations Program for HIV/AIDS), 18, 21, 29, 191
UNICEF (United Nations Children's Fund), 16, 22
United Nations: Declaration of Human Rights (1948), 38, 60; Millennium Project of, 113–114, 115. *See also* MDGs (Millennium Development Goals)
United Nations Charter: current outcomes of goals set out by, 34; peaceful coexistence rules/principles laid out in, 33
United Nations Children's Fund, 223
United Nations Coordinating Committee, 193
United States: four freedoms unifying Americans in the, 3–4; free public education mandate of, 66–68; health expenditures differences of Europe vs., 41–42; highest rates of obesity in world in, 46; life expectancy in, 38; percentage of aging workers in, 47; public health leadership development in the, 203–209; public policies on "frail elderly" in, 58
University of Cape Town, 10
University of Michigan School of Public Health, 210
U.S. Department of Agriculture, 134

U.S. National Institute for Child Health and Human Development, 45
U.S. Surgeon General, 46
U.S. Veterans Health Administration, 48
USAID (U.S. Agency for International Development), 22, 105, 108, 110, 111, 150, 210, 212, 213

V

Valkonen, T., 168
Vavilov, N., 170
Vesalius, 169

W

Walburg, P., 167
Walt, G., 202
Watt, I., 175
Wealth creation theorem, 67
Websites: "Business Principles for Countering Bribery," 98–99; Nigeria's National Agency for Food and Drug Administration and Control, 99; Public Affairs Center, 93; TI Integrity Award, 99
Webster, E., 157
Weisskopf, V., 55
White, M., 175
White, T. H., 55
Whitman, W., 7
WHO (World Health Organization): ARI case-management protocol adopted by, 223; contributions to global health by, 22, 49; Declaration of Alma-Ata by, 38; faith in science/technology solutions by, 25; on global health gap, 191; "health for all" model used by, 33, 38; health partnerships between corporations and, 29, 30; human resource development efforts by, 164; JLI (Joint Learning Initiative) work with, 149–150; on need for health system leadership, 202–203; nine principles of constitution adopted

by, 33–34; river blindness treatment collaboration with Merck, 16, 17; Soviet scientists working with, 171; study on benefits of health promotion collaboration, 131; study on inadequate health services and poverty by, 48
Winrock International, 212–213
W.K. Kellogg Program, 205
World Bank: Brazilian HIV/AIDS programs funded by, 80, 83; estimates on aging population by, 39; funding of essential health services by, 118; Global Fund to Fight AIDS role of, 27; health partnerships between corporations and, 16, 18, 22; health sector loan to Hungary by, 175; on human resources/leadership development, 149; on impact of AIDS on South Africa, 28; projections on Brazilian HIV cases by, 76, 80; public health funding to Central/ East Europe by, 179–180; World Development Report 2003 by, 151
World Bank Early Childhood Development (ECD) Virtual University, 211

World Development Report 2003 (World Bank), 151
World Economic Forum's Global Health Initiative, 22
World Health Assembly, 26
World Health Forum, 26
World Summit on Sustainable Development, 114

Y

Yen, J., 218
Yugoslavia, 172–173

Z

Zambia: "HIV/AIDS in the Workplace" program (IESC) in, 108–109; IESC Biz/AIDS program of, 105–107, 109–111; Livingstone Linkages program in, 108; SMEs (small and medium enterprises) of, 106, 107, 110, 111
Zambia Chamber of Small and Medium Business Associations, 110
Zambia District Business Associations, 110
Zatonski, W. A., 168, 180, 181
Zidovudine (AZT), 84